I0776801

A Joint Decision ... Total Knee Replacement

Your Handbook for Success

Katy Vincent

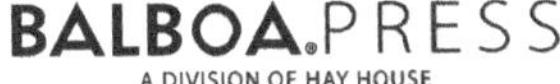

BALBOA.PRESS

A DIVISION OF HAY HOUSE

Balboa Press books may be ordered through booksellers or by contacting:

Balboa Press
A Division of Hay House
1663 Liberty Drive
Bloomington, IN 47403
www.balboapress.com.au
AU TFN: 1 800 844 925 (Toll Free inside Australia)
AU Local: (02) 8310 7086 (+61 2 8310 7086 from outside Australia)

Print information available on the last page.

ISBN: 978-1-9822-9399-4 (sc)
ISBN: 978-1-9822-9398-7 (e)

Balboa Press rev. date: 04/13/2022

CONTENTS

I wrote this book for you.

At age fifty-four, I got told by my surgeon my knee was "knackered," and I needed a brand new one.

Nine months after my knee was replaced, I was told I needed two of the lumbar joints in my spine fused and then, to top off the year of "not so great news", my surgeon told me he will probably have to replace both my hips sometime in the next ten years.

So much for our joints lasting us a lifetime!

When I got the "knackered knee" verdict, I went looking for something to help me understand what I could do to prepare for, recover from, and better manage my upcoming total knee replacement surgery. I scoured bookstores and the internet but couldn't find anything that met my requirements. This was a problem. So, I sat down and developed my own solution; and because my results were so good, I decided I should share my solution with anyone else getting a new knee. I want you to take control of your own recovery and get the best from your new knee.

I also chose to share with you some of my life experiences, the bits that slowly killed my knee, so you wouldn't end up buying a boring book of hints and empty tables.

MY ENTIRE LIFE DIDN'T GO TO PLAN, AND THAT'S OK

I knew my knee was a problem; I just didn't think I would end up with a total knee replacement this early in life. Honestly, I thought people my mum's age were the only ones that got joint replacements! She had hers done a couple of years ago, and she is eighty-two this year. It is apparant this surgery is no longer restricted to the "older" generation and more and more osteoarthritis is affecting people at an earlier age. Plus, the last twenty years have seen an increased focus on staying healthy, living longer, and being far more active as we age. Our joints are getting hammered! Not in a good way. Luckily, modern science has ways to return what osteoarthritis is taking away from us.

I have been active for most of my life, and 2020 was hard work, and not just because we were in the middle of the COVID-19 pandemic. My knee pain was so bad I couldn't exercise, go shopping or walk the dogs. Not being active was depressing and being stuck working at home for five months probably sent me a little crazy too!

Was the knee replacement verdict a surprise to me when it came? Nope. On review of my life experiences, I realised a steady stream of crazy activities completed during my adult years were the culprit. I don't regret a minute of my life so far, and on the following pages is a recap of some of my life experiences.

THE DEATH OF A KNEE

I SLID DOWN MOUNTAINS, SOMETIMES ON MY BUTT

I lived in Melbourne for about eighteen years of my adult life and had mates with ski-in/ski-out accommodation on the mountain. If there was skiable snow on the mountain, that's where you would find us on weekends. Unfortunately for my knee, my first trip to the Mt. Buller ski field (not my preferred mountain) was not a great experience. The guy next to me on the chair lift managed to tangle his snowboard under the seat just as we were trying to ski off. Being at the end of the chairlift, I tried to jump over his mess and stacked it big time! OUCH! My first ride on a snowmobile—to the medical centre—this was the first of the injuries to my right knee, and I spent a lot of that ski trip in the bar, and less time on the snow, than I had hoped for.

Back in Melbourne, at my first orthopaedic surgical consult ever, my surgeon confirmed I had torn the cartilage (aka meniscus) of my right knee and damaged the medial collateral ligament, aka MCL. The MCL healed itself after some time in a brace, as ligaments are prone to do. Alas, as my cartilage growing years were behind me; the surgeon had to cut out the tear. It wasn't large and the impact of the surgery was minimal; arthroscopic surgery has been widely adopted for knee surgeries since 1972 (thanks, Wikipedia) and leaves minimal scar tissue. This small setback didn't hold me back from the snow fields for long. The resulting trips over the years here in Australia and New Zealand involved plenty of laughs, sore muscles, and more than one hangover. I regret never going to Japan as I hear the snow there is amazing.

Peer pressure—I gave into it and got myself fitted out to try snowboarding. This was a double-edged sword. One less slippery stick stuck to my feet, but then both my feet were now stuck to a wider but shorter, and just as slippery, single stick! My first season on a snowboard was less than awesome.

First trip to snow with full snowboarding gear, ready to carve up the slopes, I caught the back edge of my snowboard on an icy run—an unrecoverable mishap—which resulted in me doing a huge "splat" backward in the middle of the trail. Given that was about my fifth fall in a row on the same run, I spat the dummy, picked up my snowboard, and stomped down the mountain in disgust. It was only after I had calmed down we realised I didn't just have a headache from banging my head on the icy slope but had also fractured my coccyx. Oops. Another trip where I spent less time on the snow than intended. I got very good at playing 500 though. Side benefit.

I CARRIED AN EXTRA 106 KG FOR TOO LONG!

I should clarify . . . I lost 20 kg of body fat and 86 kg of dead weight who we will, from now on, refer to as "the ex-boyfriend."

Other than carrying that 20 kg for way too long, how did the losing weight impact my knees?

Over nine months my programme was focussed primarily on using free weights (not machines), and I completed gazillions of dead lifts, squats, and lunges with ever-increasing weights. I calculated that in one session I had squatted the equivalent of a tonne! One thousand kilograms in forty-five minutes. That was a big legs day. My knees took the brunt of those increasingly heavier weights. My posture and technique may have been close to spot on, but the knees and the back still incur wear and tear through the process.

I WALKED 42 KM INSTEAD OF CATCHING THE BUS

January in Melbourne is awesome, and the Belgium Beer Garden in St Kilda is one of my favourites for a lazy weekend catch-up with friends. One Sunday afternoon at drinks with some friends I hadn't seen for a while, they asked me if I wanted to hike the Inca Trail with them that year, as they had a couple of spots available. My only question was—"When do we leave?"

Unlike the day tourists who jump on the train and then the bus to view the Machu Picchu ruins, our intrepid Aussie trekking team walked the trail. The Inca trail is 42 km long—the same length as a marathon—and it took us five days to walk the full length. Up the side of mountains, across valleys, and around and down more mountains, avoiding the alpacas and the llamas spitting at us.

It was the five-star version of trekking, we didn't exactly "rough it". Our Sherpas would setup for morning tea and lunch in advance of our arriving at the designated break spots, and every morning, we were roused from our tents with mugs of hot steaming cocoa and a bowl of hot water for washing up. The trail was hard work, but we were very well looked after as we wound our way along the trail.

The highest pass we went through was Dead Woman's Pass, which is 4,215 m above sea level and still 1,800 m higher than Machu Picchu. We were not up there for long, so altitude sickness wasn't an issue for us.

We had spent three days in Cusco as part of our journey so we could be a little more ready for the higher altitudes and that helped. Everyone goes through altitude adjustment differently; for me, I spent a day in bed at the hotel feeling dizzy and nauseous, but I remember a few of the guys in our group reacting as if they had smoked marijuana and were extremely stoned. Very funny to watch at the time.

I had spent four months preparing for this trek, and I recall (not fondly) doing the Kokoda Track Memorial Walk, known to Melbourne locals as the "1,000 steps," more times than I can remember. On top of all the training I did, I made sure I carried an extra 20 kg in my backpack as preparation for the trip.

I am positive someone in our group had told me we had to carry our own packs along the trail and I wanted to be prepared.

Anyway, when we got to the start of the trail, we discovered the Sherpas are super fit, altitude acclimated, and they can, and will, carry huge weights, including our backpacks, along the trail. The tips they get at the end of the trail for performing these services is a major part of their income.

Who am I to turn down a 20 kg backpack-carrying service that only cost me about US$100!

Completing the Inca Trail was physically taxing, but it was also a profoundly spiritual journey for me. My Dad had passed away the year before this trip, and the moments of solitude I sought, and found, in those mountains soothed my soul and let me say goodbye to him in my own way.

I walked away from that trip injury free and loving life. But osteoarthritis is all about wear and tear; my joints had started to incur a debt I couldn't repay with kindness.

I PIVOTED

Inspired by my own weight-loss journey, I studied part-time to obtain my personal training qualification. Newly qualified and enthused, I took a huge step sideways, and I left my project manager role to start my own business as a franchised personal trainer. I had no guarantee I would be able to match the income I had just given up, just a burning desire to help others make lasting changes to their own lives.

I loved being a personal trainer. My clients were making real changes in their lives, and I was working with other, more experienced, trainers in my gym. We had a ball trying out new and crazy exercises we would then inflict on our clients. I was seeing the benefits of my sea change, and I was loving being single, fit, and successful in my new career.

But . . . being a personal trainer was hard on my back and knees.

Remember how I had broken my coccyx snowboarding? It turned out I had other lower back issues now making themselves known to me. Loudly. When offered the opportunity to step up into the role of personal trainer manager at my gym on a secondment, I took it. This was a good decision for me physically as I was training less clients, which was better for my back, and was concentrating on recruitment and training new personal trainers, which satisfied my need to educate and train. Just in a different way.

Promoted to personal trainer manager at a sister gym, I managed to refrain from damaging my knee for a couple of years, but then, at a training master class, something went "ping" in my right knee. Again. But I did not have the time available to get the injury reviewed at the time. It wasn't until I moved back home to Perth in 2011 when I was able to make the time to see an orthopaedic surgeon about the injury. Another MRI and—OUCH—yep, I was up for another arthroscopic surgery on my right knee, just a "tidy up," but the diagnosis post-surgery wasn't great for the long-term future of my right knee.

Osteoarthritis (OA) was now evident in the joint, and my surgeon was very conscious I was young, compared to most of his other patients in the same situation, and he wanted to adopt a conservative approach to surgeries on my knee. Trying to repair every little problem in my knee was not a good option as every time he went in to "look and tidy up" meant I was one step closer to running out of cartilage.

I WAS NEARLY THROWN OFF A MOUNTAIN

Regardless of the osteoarthritis verdict, I had a life to live. Two months of working my butt off on the stepper as preparation, I dragged my—now husband—Nathan off to Nepal. Once there, we "voluntarily" completed the twelve-day Annapurna Base Camp Trek (also known as ABC Trek) with two other Aussies. After day one, Nathan was ready to throw me off the mountain, and let's face it, since I had basically "voluntold" him we were doing the trip, he probably would have gotten away with it.

This trek was hard! So much harder than doing one or two hours on the stepper at home and much harder than the Inca Trail. Maybe just because I was older. Nothing will effectively prepare you for doing 3,767 steps UP on day one. It was a physical and mental challenge to complete. We also ended up lost when we finally made it into Ghorepani, where we were staying the first night, because I was so slow. The rest of our team was already in their accommodation waiting for us to turn up by the time we made it to the front gate. It was me that was slow, not Nathan.

I thank any deity available that, once again, I had landed on a trek where we had Sherpas to carry our backpacks for tips! I could not have done that trip without their help, and even my little day bag was too much for me to carry. Backpacks sorted, all we had to worry about was the weather changes, the altitude sickness, hazardous terrain, and potential avalanches! And they say Australia is dangerous!

As we continued our ascent up the mountain, our guide pointed out a couple of areas where other avalanches had happened several years ago and remained untouched as they were still too dangerous for the bodies to be recovered from.

> *We were partway along our trek when the avalanche at Mt Everest on 18 April 2014 killed sixteen Sherpas. This was the last trek for Everest in 2014 as the Sherpas refused to work again that year in respect for the sixteen who had perished. Thirteen of the bodies were found and three remain unrecovered to this date.*

Whether we were climbing steps, walking along flat trails, or working our way down through the valleys to get to the next tea house, we did a LOT of walking. By the end of day two, my knee was telling me how very unhappy it was about this particular life choice I had made.

This trek was twelve days of "up walking," "down walking," and "slow walking"! Sujan, our crazy-fun trekking guide in Nepal had an interesting use of English to describe our itinerary each day.

Daily, we averaged between six to eight hours of hiking, and at one stage, Nathan and I debated whether I was going to need to hire a pony to take me to the base camp. I will admit, finishing the trek under my own power, had become a matter of pride for me; I didn't want to ride a pony to the base camp when I had done so much preparation for this trip. So regardless of how slow I was moving, I refused to give in and take the easy way up the mountain. I felt like it was cheating! So I persisted and by the end of day three we had learned the rhythm of the trail. Slow and steady steps for "up walking". This, my knee could cope with. The "down walking"? This was an entirely different challenge, and I cannot believe I ever wondered the value of buying hiking poles for the trek. I learned to use those trekking poles like a BOSS and it is only because of them I was able to come down those mountains under my own steam. I should have mounted them on the wall as a trophy when I got home!

The ABC Trek was one of the hardest things I have ever done, and I couldn't have done it without the other members of our trek: Nathan, the Aussies, and especially our Sherpas.

I want to thank my husband, Nathan, who gave me the moral support and encouragement I needed to get to the end of the trail on my own two feet. Without him, I would have bailed and gone back home without completing the trek, and I would have missed an amazing experience!

I JOINED A PSEUDO CULT

Back home and as recovered from the ABC Trek as I could be, I went looking for a new challenge, and I found CrossFit.

My mind was blown! How had I not found this sport before? A combination of traditional weightlifting and gymnastics. I trained alongside a super competitive and supportive group of mates who egged me on to do better at every WOD (workout of the day) I attempted. I loved this sport and did (almost) everything thrown at me! My personal best for a single dead lift was 112kg. Unfortunately, my enthusiasm was writing cheques my body couldn't cash. I couldn't do the runs, the box jumps, or any of the high impact activities; don't get me started on wall ball throws as they require deep squats my knee would complain about everytime attempted.

By now, I was wearing a knee brace for every workout and adapting all the leg exercises to adjust for my knee's limitations. I was icing my knee after each session and recovery was getting harder. I persisted and worked through my pain.

I SETTLED DOWN

Life moves on and so did we. Nathan and I got married and built our new home in a suburb some distance from where were we had been previously. Unfortunately, our new home was just too far away from my favourite CrossFit gym for me to easily attend classes.

I left my Crossfit mates behind, vowing to find an alternative. Instead of finding a new gym to workout at, we became the parents of two beautiful, but very active, fur-babies—Zeus, our Rottweiler, and Xena, our White Swiss Shepard. Now my daily exercise included training classes, walkies (sometimes twice a day), and trying not to trip over dog toys.

I HIT FITNESS ROCK BOTTOM

Without CrossFit, I was putting on the kilos, and the increasing numbers on the scales were the kick in the butt I needed to try to find something new. Taking up a Facebook advert for a free consult and first session, I started working out at Intense Health, a private studio in Perth.

Their promise was an effective workout in just twenty-minute sessions, and they delivered on this.

These workouts were effective and fitted into my working day very easily. I didn't even sweat! Full nutritional support was included in the programme, and I was enjoying this change of pace. I went alcohol free for one hundred days and in six months dropped from 30 per cent body fat to 22 per cent body fat. I felt great; I had dropped three dress sizes, and I was strong and healthy. I still appear in their adverts on Facebook from time to time.

I finally felt comfortable in my own skin again.

But my right knee was still not quite right, and we were constantly adjusting my workouts again to compensate for the pain levels in my knee. I resolved to get to my surgeon to get the pain checked out.

I made the time to go in to see my surgeon and obtained a referral for the MRI but then COVID-19 hit us. Our fitness centres and gyms closed their doors, and we were told to work from home and stay there.

Toilet paper sales went ballistic. Supermarkets became war zones, and somehow a toilet paper black market emerged as frantic Aussies tried to hoard paper. We were already subscribers to an automated service via "Who Gives a Crap," so we never ran out and in fact I could have made a profit during those months if I had been so inclined.

The pain in my knee was now constant and I couldn't even muster up the enthusiasm to workout with my equipment at home. My motivation to sweat, when I knew it would cause pain, was non-existent, and on top of that, there was the stress of the working from home for nine months and my husband being made redundant 3 months into the lockdown. Stressful times.

It is impossible for me to just sit back and do nothing for very long; enforced idleness does not sit well with me as I have been too active for too long. When life went back to being just a little bit like normal and we were allowed back into the gyms, I looked for low-impact alternative to Intense Health and I joined my local Speed-Fit studio.

A few months into this training and I realised it wasn't just impact work I couldn't do. Now I was struggling with squats, lunges, standing, walking, anything that involved putting pressure on my knee.

Pain was becoming a chronic, constant backdrop to my life.

My knee and my mental health were deteriorating at the same pace. All the work I had put in with the Intense Health crew to get healthy was gradually being reversed.

BAD DOG MUM

On top of my physical and mental decline, I was now unable to take our dogs for walks, and I felt like the world's worst dog mum. I would resort to putting them in the car and driving to a park where I could stand still and just throw the ball to them. Luckily, Zeus would retrieve and give the ball back to me to throw. If Xena got the ball, she would refuse to give it back, but at least they were getting out of the house.

We live in Perth, the most remote capital city in the world, and here in Western Australia, we have been lucky to have the lowest COVID-19 infection rates in the country due to our rigid border closures. We still had local lockdowns though, and during the pandemic, popping off to see a specialist was not an option, let alone trying to schedule an elective surgery. Appointments for MRIs and non-critical issues, such as my constant knee pain, were put on pause; however, I dug out the MRI I had obtained in January 2020, and in October, off I went to get the joint looked at.

My surgeon reviewed the MRI and was sure I needed a surgery to correct my knee issues. The only question was what "type" of surgery I needed. Another arthroscopy was booked in November for a quick "peek" at the inside of my knee. The surgeon wanted to clarify exactly what we were dealing with. I went into that surgery knowing we were looking at a full or partial knee replacement, so either verdict was not going to be a surprise.

I came out of that surgery with less cartilage and more pain! Now every step was painful; my knee felt like I was down to bone on bone.

No surprise, my surgeon confirmed my knee was riddled with osteoarthritis. There was no partial knee option; this was it. At age fifty-four, I needed a total knee replacement, and I finally I had the reason why my knee pain was so bad.

Osteoarthritis.

SURGEON PING-PONG

Being (only) fifty-four years old, my surgeon wanted me to get the most longevity out of any new knee I was the recipient of. He knew I would require a knee replacement that would give me the best possible outcome, and he referred me to one of his associates, Mr Sam Young at Perth Hip & Knee.

Sam specialises in robotically assisted knee replacements, and this was the surgery that would give me the best outcome.

I met with Sam just before Christmas, and at that session, he did not pull any punches. My knee was knackered, not at all unique, and the only thing setting me apart from his other patients was my age. I recollect he told me the damage to my knee was as common as a "barn door" and that it was a "no-brainer" to fix.

Sam replaces knackered knees like mine five days a week, every week, including public holidays. I think he does take the Christmas break off though. He assures me he can do that many because he lets the robot do all the work—I am not sure that is 100 per cent true.

Sam and his team set everything up so I could get my surgery as soon as possible in the New Year— February 2021 was the next available date. Whilst there was already a long list of surgeries planned, Sam's team said there might be opportunity to bring my surgery forward, so I got my blood tests and knee measurements done as soon as I could. I would not be the blocker if an earlier date became available.

Confirmation the hospital would open theatres for surgeries on the 25th January—the Australia Day public holiday—meant my surgery was brought forward by about three weeks. I finally had a date when I would be rid of my horrible knee pain, almost a year since I had been given the original referral for an MRI.

BRAKE LATE AND TURN

Obviously, I had known for a few years a knee replacement was going to happen at some time. I also knew the only way I was going to get a great result from my surgery was if I prepared, planned, and worked for the best possible new knee.

My personal training background has remained a solid part of my life. I missed being active, now I had a definite date for my surgery. I was now committed to preparing as best I could with what time I had left before going into the hospital.

So I hit the brakes and did an about turn—I dropped some weight, gave up drinking alcohol, and I tried to work out on my stepper at home. I wanted to go into surgery as fit and healthy as possible. I also had to plan for surgery and then recovery at home with a fly-in fly-out husband and two active (much larger now) fur babies running around the house.

I googled, I searched bookshops and newsagents, but I couldn't find the right resource. I was looking for a book or journal that would help me manage my lead up to the surgery and then allow me to plan and track my rehabilitation activities.

There were publications issued by the hospital about expectations whilst in the hospital, but nothing about everything else surrounding a total knee replacement surgery. So I resorted to using a blank notepad which I customised for my own use, and this became my bible.

I could track my medication, exercise, pain levels, appointments, and use it as reference materials at my post-surgery consults. That notepad became the blueprint for this book. This is what worked for me, and I know it can work for you too.

At my six-month post-surgery review (performance review #3), Sam told me I had the best total knee replacement recovery he has ever seen from one of his patients. I truly believe my mental, physical and logistical preparation for this surgery was a key element in my success. Sam's work on the inside of my knee and the very minimal scar I have been left with are all on him though. Thanks, Sam. 😊

WHY SHOULD YOU USE THIS BOOK?

On the following pages I have shared with you my experiences and how I planned for my own surgery and recovery; please adopt and adapt any of them that are useful for your own surgery.

There are checklists and hints, pages to plan, and pages for you to make notes on your exercises plus placeholders for recording pain levels and medication schedules. I have also provided dedicated pages for you to staple any loose documents you are given so you can keep everything in one place.

I strongly suggest you write down how your day went and make a habit of reviewing your day, and planning the next, at a set time each day. Set an alarm on your phone or smart watch if you need prompting.

These notes will help you focus any questions you may have when you go back to see your surgeon for your two-week and six-week post-surgery reviews (I will refer to these as your performance reviews). As you start working on your recovery with your physical therapist, you will want to record what exercises you are to complete and provide feedback to them on how you are managing with them.

WRITE DOWN WHAT HURTS

With everything going on in our lives, it is hard to remember what we had for dinner last Thursday night, unless it is always Mexican on Thursdays in your house. So when you get asked to describe the physical pain you experience in your knee, you may end up struggling to remember how to describe the pain. You will have even less success comparing the pains pre-surgery versus post-surgery.

Our brains are fickle things; they can remember mental pain and can recreate feelings and emotions. For example—I can recreate the pain I felt losing our beautiful Rottweiler, Zeus, by just thinking of how much I miss him. But we cannot do the same when trying to recreate the physical pain. Physical pain is an "in the moment" experience that can't be recreated on demand. The brain is amazingly good at supressing the memory of pain, and personally, I had more than a year of chronic pain in my knee, and I don't WANT to remember it.

Your turn. What were you doing this time last year that you can't do now? What activities do you struggle to complete? Go through your previous daily routine and get ready to write some initial thoughts on how you are now tracking. Don't stress if you can't remember everything now; you have until your surgery to document these.

What have you stopped doing that you loved?

Some ideas for you to get the brain going: gardening, going up and down stairs, shopping, bowls, golf, netball, basketball, football, jogging or running, riding your bike, going kayaking, rock climbing, swimming, sitting and standing.

Here is my example to help get you started—walking the dogs.

- If they pulled on the lead, this would put additional pressure on parts of my knee that were instant and extremely painful.
- My knee pain was an 8/10 at these times, and I felt like a really bad dog mum. Especially considering how fit and healthy I was two years ago.

The list below will most likely morph into being your list of what "good" would be once you have had your knee replaced. For many of us, the whole purpose of this surgery is about regaining some quality of life.

I STOPPED . . .	MY PAIN	HOW THIS MADE ME FEEL
	/10	
	/10	
	/10	
	/10	
	/10	
	/10	
	/10	
	/10	

This is your journey—be honest with yourself.

DREAMS AND GOALS—FOR YOUR KNEE

Contrary to what some people may tell you, a new knee is not going to give you super-powers. Nor will anyone be able to remotely control your knee using the garage remote or a big magnet.

Your new knee could be 90-95 per cent as good as your real knee was, IF YOU DO THE WORK. Every surgery is unique, and recovery looks different for everyone.

Your next page is your opportunity to take your "pain list" and turn it into a "happy list." Be realistic about what you want to achieve; if you never ran a marathon before, you probably won't after the surgery. That is definitely a dream, not a goal.

Share your list with your surgeon and have a chat about what is realistic. Not only can they help rationalise the goals you want to achieve, but they can also put you in contact with the right people to help you get to achieve these goals.

WHAT DOES GOOD LOOK LIKE FOR YOU?

This list is your "**Happy List.**" Every time you come back to this list and mark up that you achieved one of the goals, you should feel enthused and energised at your progress. Celebrate your successes and make sure you enjoy each goal as you achieve them.

WHAT LEVEL OF SUCCESS WILL MAKE ME HAPPY?	MONTH #	ACHIEVED BY:

HOW WILL YOU CELEBRATE YOUR SUCCESS?

PREVIOUS MEDICAL HISTORY CHECKLIST

There are a lot of things you need to provide every time you go into a surgery. If you have been extremely lucky in life, this may be your first surgery, and if that is the case, then these questions are new to you. But guaranteed you will need to recycle these multiple times during your life, so keep a hold of this book once your surgery is done. It will become good reference material.

If, like me, you have been in and out of surgery multiple times, then none of these questions are going to surprise you.

Tick off each item once completed or cross out if N/A

- ❏ Have you had a knee replacement previously?
- ❏ Have you had a poor recovery from any of them?
- ❏ Did you get any blood clots?
- ❏ Was there any excessive bleeding or bruising post-surgery?
- ❏ Do you have an existing heart problem?
- ❏ Do you have any lung problems or difficulty breathing?
- ❏ Do you suffer from a psychological or psychiatric disorder?
- ❏ Do you have gout?
- ❏ Do you have any form of diabetes?
- ❏ Do you have a history of keloid scars or poor healing after previous surgeries?

Have you had an allergy or bad reactions to any of the following?

- ❏ Anaesthetics
- ❏ Surgical tape

- ❏ Wound dressings
- ❏ Antibiotics or other medications?
- ❏ Do you have a support network at home for after the surgery?
- ❏ Have you documented all the details on all medications and supplements you are taking? Use the table provided.
- ❏ In the week prior to surgery, did you have any cuts, bites, or scratches to your legs?
- ❏ Do you have any concerns about the surgery?

If you answered Yes to any of the above questions, please make some notes below for your surgeon to review.

NOTES

"HERBS & SPICES"

I take a range of probiotics, vitamins, minerals, and fish oils as supplements daily. These are in addition to my prescribed medications, and I affectionately refer to these as my "herbs and spices."

I keep everything I have to take in a small basket stored in my scullery (next to the coffee machine), and every Sunday morning, while I am drinking my second cup of coffee, I set my week up by doling out my pills into a "Monday to Sunday" pill dispenser with my daily requirement of medications and supplements.

As I normally take these before my first coffee of each day, doing this after my Sunday coffee guarantees I am getting all the right tablets into my system during the week without having to put my brain to work too early in the day.

Now it's time to go through your "herbs and spices" basket. Write down everything you take. Doesn't matter if it is an herbal supplement or a prescribed medicine, it is all important. Make sure you also note of the dosage schedule you are on. This would be a good time to check if anything needs to be topped up (or thoughtfully disposed of if out of date).

You will need to tell the hospital when each of your medications or supplements were last taken when you go in for surgery. Be prepared to pull this list up and update it as you go into the hospital.

Your surgeon will probably ask you to stop taking products, such as fish oils and blood thinners, so make sure you follow their instructions on this matter to prevent your surgery date being compromised.

YOUR HERBS AND SPICES

MEDICATION OR SUPPLEMENT	DOSAGE/FREQUENCY	DATE LAST ONE TAKEN

MEDICATION OR SUPPLEMENT	DOSAGE/FREQUENCY	DATE LAST ONE TAKEN

If you struggle to pronounce or remember your medication names and doses—or your handwriting is so bad no-one else can read it—take a photo of the packaging as well. That way the health professionals can work out any information you may have missed.

RECIPE FOR SUCCESS

The best chefs have a team of lackeys running around their kitchen doing the preparation for guests coming to their restaurants. They plan the meals, they work out what ingredients are to be peeled and available, what meat or seafood needs to be defrosted, and plan how to get these proteins to the right temperature by time of ordering. Once you place your order, they use all of that preparation to quickly produce an amazing meal.

The level of planning and preparation the chef put into presenting you a finished, polished meal is the same recipe for success you should apply to your knee surgery.

Post-surgery infections, wound healing issues, re-admissions to the hospital, and poor results can be reduced if you are proactive in your preparation and planning.

Proper Planning and Preparation Prevents Piss Poor Performance

OWN YOUR OUTCOME

If you think you can sit back on your butt and just wait for your new knee to just magically become fully functional after your surgery, you are dreaming. You absolutely need to put some effort into ensuring your knee is going to be fully functional. In the past, that was just rehabilitation—post-surgery. You can have a better outcome if you do just a little more work before your surgery.

Become the proactive partner in this project—your surgeon can change out your knee for a new one, but if you take charge of your own preparation and recovery, you can be sure you will get the results you work for.

If YOU don't take control, you may end up disappointed in your new knee.

PREHABILITATION—A NEW CONCEPT

We know all about rehabilitation, this is the physical therapy work you do post-surgery to get better. But now let's talk about the concept of PRE-habilitation.

Prehabilitation is the work you do before you get your knee replacement. This is planning and actioning a programme of activities to ensure you go into that surgery as fit and as healthy as possible.

If you go into your surgery even just a little fitter and healthier than you are now, then you will be putting yourself into a stronger position post-surgery for a better outcome.

8 WEEKS PRE-OP—GET OFF THE COUCH

In case you missed the TV shows, the advertising and plethora of information out there, being fit and healthy is the new sexy. Regular exercise is good for you. It can help improve your sleep patterns and reduce stress levels. You might even lose some weight along the way, which could boost your self-esteem. Bonus points . . . our bodies naturally release endorphins, also known as happy chemicals, which may help reduce your pain and help you feel more relaxed in the lead-up to surgery.

It's import that you find something you can do within your current pain levels but that you also enjoy so it doesn't become a chore to complete.

Remember to check with your GP if you are new to exercise; we want you in the best shape possible for your surgery.

So why do so many people NOT go out and get some exercise? They continue to "plan" and never "do."

Because saying something and then actually doing it is hard. But so is going in for a total knee replacement, and you have already committed to one very big action AND you committed a little more by buying this book. A little bit more preparation is only going to help.

Sit down today and look at what you CAN do in the weeks or months leading up to your surgery and plan some activities. I have given you space to plan in the next couple of pages.

If you make that first step, then working your plan will get easier every day.

To keep yourself accountable:

- Partner up with a buddy who will work out with you and keep you accountable. If you don't have someone who lives locally to buddy up with, consider joining an online group or subscribe to a programme with an app on your phone to help you remain focussed.
- Book activities you have to pay for, that also have a cancellation charge if you don't turn up; no-one likes to lose money.
- Put your plan up on the fridge as well as in here.
- Schedule it in your phone or write it in your diary.

You absolutely CAN find thirty mins a day to do something that makes you sweat, and the most important part of that activity is getting off the couch and just doing it. Overcoming inertia is the hardest part of an exercise programme.

Here are some ideas for you if you need inspiration.

- Find a Pilates studio near you (they do small, supervised classes).
- Borrow, rent, or buy an exercise bike (great for rehabilitation) or a rowing machine or get to a gym that has this equipment. You can get gym memberships on weekly or casual memberships.
- Find a pool centre close by where you can use the lap-pool. Hydro/Aqua classes are a great way to get fit whilst not making your knee angry (and you can make new friends).
- Do some resistance training, increase strength in your arms and legs. Remember you are going to be using a walker or crutches for a little while.

If you need help, see a physiotherapist, physical therapist, personal trainer, or a gym near you. They can help you work out what prehabilitation exercises are most appropriate for you.

WHAT ACTIVITIES CAN I DO NOW?

Have a look around now at some activities in your area; make enquiries about attending the right classes or getting access to the right trainer at your gym or recreation centre for support.

Jot down some notes about what you have found that you might like to try out, and find out what they can offer you.

Tip—If you can't do the thirty minutes all at once, then try to split your efforts across two or even three sessions in your day. So long as you can accumulate thirty minutes of exercise in your day, you will be making progress.

PREPARATION AND PLANNING

Have you decided what activity or activities you are going to try? You don't have to stick to just one; you can swap and change if a particular activity is not working for you.

As you work your way through the weeks leading up to surgery, keep track of how you are feeling. Are you getting stronger?

Do the workouts feel like they are getting easier? Use the smiley faces to check in at the end of each week.

PLAN	WEEK 1	WEEK 2	WEEK 3	WEEK 4
ACTIVITY				
PLANNED				
DONE				
UPDATE	☺ 😐 ☹	☺ 😐 ☹	☺ 😐 ☹	☺ 😐 ☹
PLAN	WEEK 5	WEEK 6	WEEK 7	WEEK 8
ACTIVITY				
PLAN				
DONE				
UPDATE	☺ 😐 ☹	☺ 😐 ☹	☺ 😐 ☹	☺ 😐 ☹
PLAN	WEEK 9	WEEK 10	WEEK 11	WEEK 12
ACTIVITY				
PLAN				
DONE				
UPDATE	☺ 😐 ☹	☺ 😐 ☹	☺ 😐 ☹	☺ 😐 ☹

Breaking a habit takes as long as it takes, don't give up trying

NUTRITION

A healthy immune system will help prevent infection from the inside. Try to focus on getting lots of vegetables, fresh fruits, and lean proteins onto your plate in the lead-up to your surgery and during recovery. Eating foods rich in protein, antioxidants, and vitamins such as C and D will push your body into a higher gear.

As you work through your prehabilitation exercise programme, you may find you are already craving healthier foods. This is the body reinforcing your great decision and asking you to get the right nutrition into your system as preparation for surgery.

There are many companies who will prepare all healthy food for you. Twenty years ago healthy didn't always mean tasty; thankfully, that definitely changed. I will talk more about these later in the book as there are options that don't involve you doing any cooking prior to going into the hospital.

This is an opportunity to try something different.

KEEP YOUR DIABETES UNDER CONTROL

If you know you already have diabetes, Type I or II, then I shouldn't need to remind you to look after yourself. If your diabetes is not well controlled before and after surgery, then this increases the risk of complications with your knee replacement surgery.

Your results will be better if your diabetes is under control. Don't give your family and friends the opportunity to yell at you for not looking after yourself. Take control now so you get the best result you can and make sure you consult with your GP or specialist if you need your condition re-evaluated.

QUIT SMOKING NOW

It's a given, smokers have a higher risk of infections and complications due to the toxins cigarettes leave in our bodies and the long-term effects of these, and nicotine, on our immune system. Pretty sure there are a gazillion reasons why you shouldn't smoke, and telling you to quit is easy. There are plenty of good reasons to quit now, including the benefits to your health.

Recovery from your surgery may be impacted by your smoking, and the best thing you can do for you is work out how to reduce or completely quit smoking. Hospitals do not put convenient smoking areas around the hospital, and rarely are these areas situated right outside your ward or room. Keep in mind you are going to have to get up and go to a distant area to smoke if you haven't quit. The flip side, if you quit too late, you are going to have to go cold turkey when you go into the hospital. Recovering from knee surgery is hard enough without throwing quitting smoking into that equation.

I am in no way qualified to give you advice on quitting smoking. Yes, I quit smoking after two failed attempts more than twelve years ago. But my story is not yours and not indicative of what your success might look like.

If you want to stop and you need help to quit or reduce your smoking, talk to your GP about a solution that works for you and give yourself sufficient time in advance so you are not going through the initial withdrawals when you go in for your surgery.

There is very little information about the effect of medicinal cannabis on your surgery or recovery; please consult with your surgeon if you are currently using any of these products.

DENTAL / SKIN CHECKS / PODIATRY WORKS

No one ever thinks that little things such as an infected tooth or toenail might put your knee surgery in jeopardy. But any infection in the six months post knee surgery may cause your body to divert much needed resources, that might be working on healing your knee, to an infection somewhere else in your body. Or worse, drag the infection from your tooth down into your new knee, which is already fighting for its own survival.

If you are due for any non-knee related appointments in the six months after your surgery, try to bring them well forward in your planning so you get there before your surgery. That way, if there are any works that need to be done around these appointments, like fillings, root canal work, or ingrown toe surgery, these are sorted out well prior to your surgery.

Post-surgery infections can jeopardise all the hard work you have already completed in your prehabilitation.

SPECIALTY MEDICAL CLEARANCE(S):

If you have any medical conditions that could impact your surgery and recovery, please make an appointment with your specialist as early as possible to discuss your upcoming knee surgery with them.

You will need clearance from your specialists prior to your surgery and will need to take these with you to one of your pre-surgery consults. Some specialists have a long waiting list, even when you are an existing patient, so get in early and make that appointment.

Fill in the table provide with all your specialist details so you have them all in one spot. Staple each of your written clearances into this book so your surgeon can take a copy if you don't have an electronic version you can email to them.

MY SPECIALIST DETAILS

SPECIALIST DETAILS	APPOINTMENT DATE	CLEARED FOR SURGERY?

LEGAL STUFF

I am not being a pessimist, and to be honest, I only got around to doing these things just last month—well after my own knee surgery—but these are a couple of boxes you should tick as part of "life" if you haven't already.

Organise, or update, the following documents before your surgery and make sure your family is aware of the location of the documents, if you don't have a lawyer that holds these for you.

- ❏ Your Will
- ❏ Power of Attorney
- ❏ Your Advanced Health Directive
- ❏ Organ Donation registration
- ❏ Your important paperwork, like life-insurance policies
- ❏ Passwords to your crypto wallet (just kidding—they should be in the safe)

NEVER WORK WITH KIDS OR PETS

As a dog mum, the one thing I stressed most about was "how do I walk my dogs" after my knee surgery. It's not like I was going to be able to drive anywhere, as I was doing pre-surgery when my knee was super sore, and then just throw the ball from the driver's seat! After surgery, I still had six weeks before my surgeon was going to let me start driving my car again. Until then, I would have to rely on my husband (if he was not working) and visiting family members to help me out by walking the dogs over the first six weeks post-surgery.

There are options.

If you plan to put your best friends into a boarding kennel, and you haven't already called them, you may have to call in a favour or two, but now is the time to book your pets into your preferred location.

If you are not boarding your pets, you may have a friend or relative who can help out. If not, you could look at engaging a pet walking service.

If you are engaging a pet walker, regardless of who they are, make sure both your pets and the pet walker have some positive experiences together and are comfortable with each other before you head off to surgery. Some ideas:

- ☐ Have the pet walker come with you on your planned walks for a week or two before surgery.
- ☐ Make sure your pet walker has practiced a solo walk with your pets—have them come to the house when you are not home, let themselves in, greet the pets, and take them for a walk, then come back to the house, follow the normal post-walk routine, and lock up the house. You want to be sure your pets are comfortable with the routine and the pet walker.
- ☐ Consider having time locks installed on your front door.
- ☐ Consider having a camera installed on your front lobby so that you can confirm the pet is home safely and the house is locked up.
- ☐ Buy some amazing new toys for the pets and let the dog walker know where they are so they can be revealed when they need your pets to be distracted and happy.

I sent our dogs away to my friend's place in Moora where they had five acres to run around in. Actually, I think they resented coming home after so many rabbits to chase. But having them not in the house meant I could recover knowing I was being the best dog mum possible.

PET FOOD—ON DEMAND OR IN BULK

If you are not sending your pets to a boarding kennel, you will want to make sure you have enough pet food on hand.

You can organise for dog food to be delivered to your home during the six to eight weeks post-surgery. Alternatively, if you have sufficient space, you could order their favourite meals in bulk and store them in the freezer.

YOUR CHILDREN CAN HELP

Depending on their ages, your kids are the best of helpers. If you need ice, water, or even a coffee, they are almost always happy to help out; you just need to make sure they return your crutches when you need them, or you might find them scattered across the house.

5 WEEKS PRE-OP

PREHABILITATION OF YOUR HOME

Just like you are preparing your body for surgery, your house probably needs to be surgery ready too.

Whilst home is totally suitable for you now, whilst you are still pretty mobile, when you start wandering around the house with walking aids, you will most likely change your mind about its suitability.

Take the time now; be proactive and make sure you ensure there are no hazards that may cause you injury or inconvenience when you are back home.

Below is a list of changes you can make to ensure your house has been prepared for your return home after surgery.

GETTING YOUR HOME READY FOR YOUR RETURN:

☐ Install a toilet at a comfortable height for you during your rehab.
You can buy or hire a seat that goes over your toilet that is higher than your normal toilet so you don't have to bend so far. New knees don't like bending.

☐ Install a horizontal and/or vertical grab bar on the walls beside the toilet.
If you are hiring a comfort seat, make sure it has the rails attached.

☐ Get a shower seat for your shower.
You can rent one or buy a plastic garden chair from your local hardware company. Install horizontal and/or vertical grab bars for the shower if your shower seat does not have one.

☐ Clear pathways for easy movement on crutches.
Move furniture and tripping hazards to ensure you have a path wide enough for mobility equipment to pass through.

☐ Check power cords to prevent trips.
Secure them to the floor with tape if they are required.

☐ Remove rugs and slippery carpets.
Falling on your butt when your crutches slide out from under you unexpectedly—ouch!

☐ Install nightlights down dark hallways and next to your bed.
It's not fun fumbling for your crutches in the dark!

☐ Set up an easily accessible "nesting" space with furnishings such as: a comfortable recliner with arms, a day bed, your cold therapy unit, a mini fridge to keep drinks ice cold, power boards to support electronics and chargers, a tool for grabbing things, etc.

❏ Place commonly used items at waist height to prevent the need to squat or bend.

❏ If you don't have a clothes drier, or it's at ground level, get a drying rack for your laundry.

❏ Organise a gardener if necessary for at least six weeks.
I still couldn't do gardening for another three months after I ditched the crutches.

❏ Have someone check your house security.

❏ Pause any scheduled deliveries while you are in the hospital.
Nothing yells "rob me—I am not home" more effectively than a pile of unread newspapers at the front door.

❏ Organise for your letterbox to be cleared or mail held at the Post Office.

❏ Have a cleaner come in on a regular basis to help keep your house under control.

DID YOU COME UP WITH ANY OTHERS?

YOUR SUPPORT PERSON

You might think you can do it all by yourself (certainly my mum tries to do it all herself), but you actually do need a support person by your side, even if just so you can whinge to them about the traffic delays on the way to an appointment.

Your support person maybe your partner, son or daughter, or a friend or case/social worker. They will be someone you trust to help you during this period.

Your support person is there to help you do what you can't do by yourself, some examples might be:

- They (might) cook your meals, put out the rubbish bins, water your plants, and answer the door for Uber Eats.
- Make sure you do your exercises and take your pain medications at the right time.
- Provide transport to and from appointments. You could take an Uber or other ride share service if you want, but sometimes it's nice to chat to someone along the way.
- Stay with you for a few days after you return home to help you organise everything you might need at the couch.
- They can pop to the shops for stuff you have forgotten.
- They can also be your second set of ears at appointments. Sometimes we only hear half of what is going on because we are in pain, distracted, or English may be our second language. Don't stress, your support person can help fill in any gaps in understanding later.
- Be there to hold your hand and talk to you about how you are feeling, physically and emotionally.

Sometimes it might actually be easier to have someone OTHER than your partner as your support person. I will let you be the judge of that decision.

FALL ALARMS

Mum was going home to an empty house after her (last) hip replacement, so my sisters organised a fall alarm for her. This was for our peace of mind, not hers. You might like to look into organising a similar system if you are going home to your own company so your family will be notified if you have a fall at home and can respond accordingly.

Please follow the directions for the device. These were written with your safety, and your family's stress levels, in mind.

Real story—an elderly member of our family was required to wear a fall alarm after a fall resulting in a quite serious back injury. She was told she could only put her device on charge when someone was with her, and she agreed to this condition. A couple of weeks later, she put her device on charge and went to bed, mobile on silent and leaving her device on charge overnight on the kitchen bench. At 3 a.m., her device, having recorded her as being in one place for too long, had activated the fall alarm parameters and sent off multiple alarms to family members whose increasingly more panicked phone calls to her mobile were not being answered.

Luckily, in this case, all ended well, and whilst our family member was not impressed at being woken at 4 a.m. by emergency services, she probably took ten years off the expected life span of her kids before they were notified there was no emergency.

There are rules that need to be followed, so please don't alarm your family unnecessarily.

Some local councils can provide you with a subsidised fall alarm; your pharmacy or your GP should be able to point you in the right direction to find a device best for your circumstances.

The fall alarm technology differs across countries. They will use one of your local carrier services to communicate via 4G or 5G or by Bluetooth to your phone.

If you need technical help, ask one of the grandkids to help!

3 WEEKS PRE-OP

PREOPERATIVE MEDICAL CLEARANCE

Everyone is different; your surgeon may request you provide a written clearance for surgery from your GP if you are at risk. This might include routine lab monitoring, and if necessary, they will recommend more testing to evaluate certain heart or lung conditions. You should organise this visit several weeks before your surgery. Not just so that any medical issues or tests can be quickly addressed but so you have sufficient lead time to get in to see the specialists.

It seems like every medical service I have had to use in the last twelve months has long lead time for getting appointments.

PRE-OP SURGICAL CONSULT

Your surgeon's team should make a booking for you to go back in to see your surgeon one to two weeks prior to surgery. It may be a phone consult or an in-person visit. At this session, your surgeon will want to review the medical clearance from your GP and any other specialist medical recommendations or clearances you have obtained.

You will be required to provide some blood samples. Blood work is required as part of your preparation for a knee surgery, and your surgeon will review the lab work and discuss with you their findings if there are any risks identified.

Make sure you bring your list of questions (plus your support person) with you to this appointment. The amount of detail you could receive in response to your questions may be more than you can easily remember.

QUESTIONS?

Remember how I said your surgeon may want you to stop taking fish oils and blood thinners? Time to remember that advice and stop taking them (if you haven't already done so). Also, maybe check in with your chemist and get a couple of your standard scripts filled so you have a buffer of supplies at home.

BTW: Aspirin is also a blood thinner, so if you have been taking it, stop now, if you haven't already.

PREPARE OR ORDER HEALTHY FOOD

During your recovery, you won't really want to be on your feet doing cooking. If you have a partner or family member who can cook fresh meals for you, then you are sorted; however, you may have to look at other options.

Take this opportunity, before surgery, to try out some of the pre-prepared meals that you can buy online from Youfoodz, My Muscle Meals, or Weight Watchers. It all depends on what's available in your area. Keep an eye out for discount deals or referral codes that can help you keep costs low whilst you try out a couple of offerings.

These companies will deliver your order to your front door on your preferred days. The boxes they deliver your meals in will be insulated and probably contain ice packs, so if you are not home when they are delivered, they will not spoil before you can get them into the fridge. Plan the deliveries in advance so you know exactly what days they will turn up at your home and watch your phone for the SMS notifications of delivery.

Don't fail to check their delivery notification. Check that they have delivered your food to YOUR front door. I have just recently had a delivery go to Avonly Cres rather than Cranberry Cres because the courier was too lazy to check Google. The photo of my meal box sitting at someone else's front door was my first clue!

Some of the meals can be stored in the fridge or freezer. With all the services I have used, my meals are able to be reheated in the microwave and still taste great! I don't even bother getting a plate out for some of my meals (keeps the dish washing requirements low).

If you get tired of the prepacked meals, install an online fresh food delivery app on your phone or bookmark a site on your computer so you can order the occasional meal in. Contactless delivery means they will leave your meal at the door. Bonus—you don't have to try to bolt to the front door to meet them!

SKIN HEALTH

The older we are the less collagen we have in our skin and the more fragile our skin becomes. I have no suggestions on how you might stop that happening—that's outside of my pay grade—but what you can do is prepare your skin for surgery. What does "prepare" mean in this scenario?

This means doing your best to stay injury free prior to surgery and that you grab some moisturiser (not the partner's best face cream; we want you alive for surgery) and apply to your legs at least once a day for a minimum of two weeks before your surgery date.

It always amazes me that when I get out into the garden, it is guaranteed I will end up with scratches on my hands and legs. If any of these scratches and nicks had become even slightly infected, that small thing could have delayed my surgery.

Your skin acts as a physical barrier to infection, so it follows that healthy and intact skin on your legs lowers the chance of infection post-surgery.

7 DAYS PRE-OP

YOUR MEDICAL AIDS – THE GOOD, THE BAD & THE UGLY

Having the right equipment ready for you at home is super important. You may have to order your own walker, cane, and crutches (our family has a history of hip, knee, and back issues, so I just get mine from Mum when I need them), but most medical equipment suppliers allow you to order online, and you can usually hire direct from the hospital pharmacy.

I recommend you make use of the online facility, if you are unable to visit in person, and choose the equipment you want in advance as they will deliver to your house and install too, if required.

You can also hire or purchase your medical aids from your local chemist or mobility provider. Here is a list of things you might need:

- Crutches
- Walking frame
- Walking frame with wheels + seat
- Elevated over-toilet seat
- Shower chair

- Non-slip shower mat, high-back day chair with adjustable height legs
- Long-handled shoe-horn
- Pick-up grasper/reacher

CRUTCHES

You should take your crutches for a test drive so you are not trying to learn a new skill straight after a big surgery. If you have never used crutches before, it's not something you will enjoy learning "on the fly." Depending on your current mobility, you may be using a walker instead of crutches.

My mum has extensive experience in this area, and below are a couple of her observations.

Once you get mobile on your crutches and are ready to face the world, how are you going to manage your handbag? Using crutches means both hands are fully occupied, and if you are trying to walk around AND carry a handbag at the same time, it is a disaster. So you look for alternatives.

- *A bag slung over your shoulder—it slips off and down your arm.*
- *Over the body—you cannot put very much into it, and it flops into the crutches when moving.*
- *A bum bag (aka fanny pack) is too small and only holds your wallet, phone, and keys.*

What are you left with? A backpack.

Your hands are now free to manage your crutches; your posture improves, especially if you put your milk, bread, and magazines in it when you go to the shops.

Crutches are the herald that precedes you when you are out in public—it is immediately obvious you have an injury and should be avoided.

It's easy to get around quickly once you have the hang of them. Getting up and down stairs is a challenge initially, but once you get the "good leg to heaven, bad leg to hell" habit and co-ordination sussed, you are good to go.

You just can't carry anything around the home without making a mess—try getting your coffee from the kitchen to the lounge room using crutches! In addition to that challenge, your arms get sore, your abs take a hiding, and they always fall over when you are sitting at a café. Why is it you can never get them on your arms fast enough, and if you do, they are on the wrong arms!?

Don't get me started on trying to get them organised when you need to go to the toilet in the middle of the night and you are trying not to step on the cat, the dog, or the husband!

WALKING FRAME

A walking frame is great if you just can't manage the crutches, but it still has to be lifted and moved by you, so you need to make sure it is nice and light, so you don't end up feeling like you are doing a gym workout every time you have to move somewhere.

I liked having this available to me at night, as I could put it close to the bed and it didn't disappear every time I had to get out of bed—unlike my crutches that seem to have a mind of their own at night. Also doesn't matter if you grab it back to front, it will wait for you to get organised.

Probably not great for carrying coffee to your home office or lounge, but still a useful aid at home.

WALKER WITH WHEELS AND A SEAT

These can be a bit hard to handle if you are on your own and are still putting all your weight on just one leg.

But depending on where you are during your recovery, they are a good choice for social outings. There is a convenient seat you sit on, literally anywhere, if your friends are taking forever to make a shopping decision. Plus, you can put a box under the seat for your valuables and hang a basket on the front for your purchases, freeing up your hands for the walker.

Getting up and down stairs is not easy with a walker on wheels—unless it is nice and light. You may need to find the closest travelator, or lift, and you should definitely practice co-ordinating the brakes with your forward movement at home well before heading out into retail world.

At home this is a slightly better option than the crutches, as it pushes the cats, dogs, and the husband out of the way when you are in control. Remember to use the brakes at the right times so it doesn't scoot out of reach just as you need it. During the day, you can put another small basket on the seat on your walker where you can put your coffee, snacks, phone, and medications and move around the house without making a mess or having to ask for as much assistance.

ELEVATED OVER-TOILET SEAT

Unless you can already do one legged squats (very difficult exercise for 99 per cent of us) before your surgery, you will need some assistance getting on and off the toilet. The arms on the over-toilet seat make this task much easier. Bending your knee whilst sitting on the "throne" is not really an achievable goal in the first few weeks you are home; it takes a bit of time before you get to that point. I don't suggest you plan to spend extended time in the toilet unless you have the over-toilet seat to help you get back up again.

SHOWER CHAIR + NON-SLIP SHOWER MAT

When I told one of my work mates I had a shower chair for the first six weeks of my recovery, she was highly amused and declared that I wasn't eighty, surely I could stand in the shower on my own?

But you know what? I can't stand on one leg in the shower for an extended period when I have two good knees ready to take up the slack. Trying to shower on one leg when the other knee is not available to me—if I have a wobble, I am a goner. How do you manage if you drop the soap? The shower chair is the obvious smart choice, and it allows you some security from slipping and landing on your butt whilst showering.

Safety Warning (again), crutches will slip on wet tiles, so invest in a couple of non-slip shower mats. Not the kind your mum put in the bottom of your bath when you were a kid (yes, you can still buy these), but there are some very cool clear pebble like mats available (Bunnings and Spotlight have them here in Australia) that look nice and work a treat.

HIGH-BACKED CHAIR

I hired a high-backed chair for use at home for a couple of weeks, I was often on my own as my hubby is a "fly-in fly-out" worker. Which means he is not always available to help me in and out of the lounge, so the chair was easiest to get in and out of unassisted.

When I could get myself out of the lounge without assistance, it was a no brainer for me to move across to there and spread out. Hubby was great and made me a custom table that surrounded the lounge on two sides. It was just the right size to hold my cold therapy device, phone, water, pain medications, books, and any other paraphernalia I thought I needed—including a bell so I could let him know every time I needed his assistance. I wonder what happened to that bell; I don't think I have seen it for a while . . .

SHOEHORN & REACHER

You won't be able to bend your knee far enough to put shoes on unless you are super flexible. The shoe horn you choose should be the right length for your leg and arm reach. If you are a tall guy using a 20 cm shoe horn and getting your shoes or socks on will be an extraordinary feat and worth taking a video of, IF you actually manage to get your shoes on.

The mobility store will have a range of lengths for you to choose from.

The Reacher, my favourite helper after the over-toilet seat. It let me pick up clothes, dropped phones, and remotely steal chips from my husband's snack plate. It can translate into a useful tool in everyday life, even after you are off the crutches (my mum uses it to pick up lemons from under her tree).

5 DAYS PRE-OP

YOUR TRANSPORT

You won't be cleared to drive for approx. six weeks after the surgery, so you will need to find alternative solutions:

- Get familiar with your local ride share provider and install the app onto your phone; they are reliable, easy-to-use, and you don't need to carry cash with you.
- Ask family/friends/support person to be available as drivers. Remember they will do their best but may get a bit tired of driving you around after a while, so share the task around or be prepared to use your ride share app occasionally.
- Taxis are always an option if you can't get a ride share service near you.

I DO NOT recommend public transport for the first 8 weeks post surgery. You are too likely to be bumped around.

MOTOR VEHICLE INSURANCE COVER

Motor Vehicle Insurance companies in Australia have the right to refuse to cover you and your property if you have an accident driving your car before your surgeon clears you for this activity.

Please check with your own motor vehicle insurance provider to confirm what they require to reinstate your cover post-surgery.

PRE-ADMISSION PHONE CALL

The hospital admission process is pretty solid; let's face it, admitting patients is a process they have been working on for a while.

You can guarantee your pre-admissions department will call you to make sure you know the important things to remember to bring with you.

The hospital will ask you a series of questions that, hopefully, you have already written down answers for earlier this book.

2 DAYS PRE-OP

PACKING FOR THE HOSPITAL

Two days to go. Time to do a practice run for your trip to the hospital.

How much do you plan to take to the hospital? The following list and tips may not be exactly to your requirements, but hopefully, it is a good start.

Don't be afraid to take some things you won't have access to in the hospital; I took my own pillow as I get a sore neck from hotel and hospital pillows. I also took my own cold therapy machine for use post-surgery (I will talk about that later), my favourite snuggle rug as it rolled up and is very small, plus a couple of warming hand packs to put into my bed whilst I was waiting to go into surgery. The nurses are always happy to get you additional heated blankets during your wait, but it gets very cold in the pre-surgery waiting room!

THE "YOU ARE NOT GOING ON A HOLIDAY" PACKING

No more than three days in the hospital including your day of surgery? Keep it simple. Make sure the clothes you wear to the hospital are suitable to wear when you leave and you can get away with just a small overnight bag for your clothes and a separate bag for your snuggle rug and other physical therapy devices.

Going in for a bit longer, just pack a couple of extra shirts and underwear.

CLOTHES

- Loose pyjamas or short sleeping shirt—I love buying some new PJ's to take to the hospital as a small treat for myself
- Under garments—comfortable ones!
- Bed Socks—if you suffer from cold feet
- Summer—loose-fitting shorts. Remember, they have to get over your knee dressing.
- Winter—Sweatpants or jogging pants, also loose-fitting
- Weather appropriate t-shirt, top, and/or front-fastening jumper (aka cardigan, pullover, sweatshirt, jersey, etc. for the non-Aussies)
- Non-slip footwear that is easy to put on and remove that won't fall off when you leave the hospital on crutches or if using a walking frame.

PERSONAL ITEMS

- Electronics: Mobile phone with charger, iPad or tablet, laptop, etc.
- Personal toiletries,
  - Toothbrush (tip—don't take the rechargeable, go old-school; there is naff all-bench space in the hospital bathroom).
  - Deodorant.
  - Skin Care—what is the very least you can get away with whilst in the hospital? You won't have the time or the energy to stand up in the tiny bathroom to go through a seven-step skin regime twice a day. Take some face cleansing wipes and your favourite night-time moisturiser and treat the visit like an extended moisturising session.
  - Electric or other razor + shaving cream IF you can't deal with the itch for more than two days.
  - Comb, Chapstick, any other cosmetics you absolutely cannot go without. NO powders allowed though.
- Books, kindle, magazines, pen & (don't forget) this book!

MEDICAL EQUIPMENT & AIDS

- Glasses—leave the contacts at home
- Hearing aid and batteries
- CPAP machine settings, tubing, and machine
- Crutches (if you have organised beforehand)

** Do not bring your walker unless you are specifically advised to do so.*

Hospitals are not banks, and whilst they will provide some security for small things—a lockable drawer—don't pack valuables such as jewellery, credit cards, or large amounts of cash. You "might" want some small amounts of cash to buy coffee or magazines, but almost all services will accept a credit or debit card payment type.

ADDITIONAL ITEMS YOU WANT TO TAKE WITH YOU

ALLERGIES

The hospital and the nurses are going to ask you multiple times what you are allergic to. Take the time now to note your allergies so you can just show them the book if required.

ALLERGY	RESPONSE

DOCUMENTS YOU SHOULD TAKE TO THE HOSPITAL

- ☐ Copy of your Advanced Directives
- ☐ Power of Attorney (if required)
- ☐ Driver's license or photo ID, insurance card, Medicare or Medicaid card
- ☐ Private Health Insurance details
- ☐ Veterans Card
- ☐ Pension/Concession card / Safety Net card or Seniors Health card
- ☐ Motor Vehicle Claim details
- ☐ Workcover Claim details
- ☐ Your GP details
- ☐ Cardio Card
- ☐ All relevant x-rays, scans, etc.

Each country is different—check with your hospital for the definitive list of documents you should take with you.

<table>
<tr><td>WHAT DID I MISS?</td></tr>
<tr><td>

</td></tr>
<tr><td>

</td></tr>
<tr><td>

</td></tr>
</table>

MY CONTACT LIST

If you are like me, ALL your contacts are stored in your mobile phone, and that is of no use if your mobile is temporarily lost somewhere in your luggage, turned off, flat (left the charger at home?), or password protected.

Rather than have everyone around you stressing about who your contacts are, why not jot down any important contact names and numbers below. Also, this way, you also don't have to teach someone how to use your mobile phone.

Don't forget to put some context against the contact name—eg, best friend, husband, heart specialist, etc. Just makes it a little easier to work out who that person is to you.

CONTACT NAME	PHONE NUMBER

24 HOURS PRE-OP

DRESS REHEARSAL

Ok. Your mobility equipment is sorted, your home living space is tidied up/locked down/converted for you using a walking aid, your pets are sorted, and your transport booked. It's time to get you ready to go to the hospital.

I try to do a dress rehearsal of my bag pack and then live out of it for twenty-four hours. If I have missed something it becomes very clear what needs to be added to my bag, including upsizing, or downsizing, my luggage.

Check your benches when you have finished packing. Have you left anything out you will need during your hospital stay?

DOUBLE & TRIPLE CHECK YOUR LIST

It never hurts to go through your check list again, but remember, you always have your support person (and access to the internet) if you forget something.

If you are a checker of lists, here is your day before surgery check list . . .

- ☐ I have organised someone to take me to the hospital.
- ☐ I have organised for someone to pick me up when I am ready to go home.
- ☐ I have arranged for someone to stay with me after I get home.
- ☐ I have told my family, friends, and work about my operation and booked my time off with HR.
- ☐ I have organised someone to look after my home and collect my mail until I get back (or stopped my mail at the Post Office—people still get snail mail?).
- ☐ I have organised help with housekeeping.
- ☐ I have pre-habilitated my home for my return.
- ☐ I have organised food delivery or prepped enough meals for two weeks.
- ☐ I have cancelled my home help and Meals on Wheels while in the hospital.
- ☐ I have medically prepared for my surgery.
- ☐ I have left all valuables safely at home rather than bring them into the hospital.
- ☐ I have packed clothes as per my previous list and have easy to put on shoes.
- ☐ I am ready for my surgery!

FINAL PREPARATION

Depending on your hospital, the following may change slightly, but regardless, the following are a list of things I was advised I needed to do before surgery. They make sense to me.

YES

- Remove any nail polish.
  - *The surgical team need to see your finger nails so they can confirm circulation during surgery. Bright red talons make that challenging.*
- Sleep in clean pyjamas or clothes.
  - *Given you probably showered with the antibacterial wash they suggested, dirty PJs or sheets would just negate the value of that effort.*
- Sleep on freshly laundered sheets.
- Confirm that your ride to the hospital knows your schedule.

o *You don't need extra stress on the day of surgery; give yourself plenty of time to be at the hospital.*
- Shower the morning of surgery using the provided or recommended antibacterial soap and wash your hair with it if advised to do so.

NO

- Don't have a big night on the eve of surgery.
  - *No one wants you to go into the hospital with a hangover and oozing alcohol from your pores.*
- Don't eat or drink anything after the time you were instructed.
  - *That includes ice chips, gum, or mints.*
- Don't smoke or vape.
  - *I hope you already quit this habit; that this is something you can virtually high-five yourself for doing.*
- Don't use lotions or powders on face or body.
- Don't shave before surgery—anywhere.
- Don't shower the morning of your surgery unless you have been advised to do so and only with the antibacterial soap recommended.
- Don't take your insulin, unless otherwise instructed.
- Don't take any of your medications or supplements on the morning of your surgery *unless otherwise instructed.*

Please re-read any materials supplied to you by your doctor or the hospital to make sure you have covered all the specific requirements specified by your surgeon or hospital.

DID I MISS ANYTHING YOU HAVE TO DO?

ANESTHESIOLOGY CONSULT

Your anaesthetist should have made an appointment to discuss your surgery either face-to-face or by phone or teleconference. During this discussion they should have checked how you responded to anaesthetics taken during previous surgery, what pain killers you may have used post-surgery previously, and how you reacted to them. They will also check what allergies you may have, your height and weight, and provide you with the opportunity to ask questions if you are not sure of something.

Once you are in the hospital, they will check in with you again, either before you get taken down to surgery or in the surgical waiting room.

ANTICIPATED LENGTH OF STAY

Most of us can go home after one to three days, and some are actually able to leave the same day as surgery. It depends on how well you have prepared and, in other cases, where you are to be released to after surgery.

The criteria for going home include:

- You are comfortable on oral pain medications.
- You are holding down food and water.
- Your bladder and bowels are properly working (some pain medications block you up, so this is important).
- You are medically stable.
- You have had your wound checked and dressing changed.
- Physical therapy has cleared you as safe to leave.
- Your support person is there to take you home.

No one likes being in the hospital for too long, but in some cases, if you are going home to an empty house, you may be kept in for a little longer. I was able to leave after three days but only because my husband was able to look after me at home. My mum stayed in two extra days as she was going home to her own company.

You will feel better at home with your own things around you, and it does make it easier to get back to a normal routine if you don't have an extended stay at the hospital. Plus the beds are JUST not comfortable.

Most of us are lucky enough to go directly home after surgery, and we don't need to go to a rehabilitation or skilled nursing facility before then.

But everyone is different, and if you do need additional support, Social Services at the hospital can arrange for visiting nurses and therapists to come into your home once you go home and work with you on recovery and rehabilitation. Make sure you have researched what options you have. If you have private health, some of them will cover the costs around these services.

POST SURGERY

PAIN MANAGEMENT

Your first couple of days after surgery at the hospital will be intense. For me, I had a nerve block plus long-acting pain relief as part of my surgery, plus I am pretty sure they pumped some additional pain relief into my knee so I was not in pain for the first twenty-four hours post-surgery. After that, your pain levels will be managed by oral pain relief. This will be managed by your anaesthetist, in consultation with you and your surgeon.

If you have had a bad reaction to any pain medications previously, this should have been discussed with your team prior to the surgery. Personally, I can't take codeine-based pain relief as it makes me super nauseous, so make sure you let your team know if you have a similar experience with anything. A gentle reminder that some pain killers can cause constipation, and until you have a bowel movement, your surgical team is not going to release you from the hospital. I sometimes think that might be the hardest bit about leaving the the hospital. It can be a tricky goal to achieve.

Same day as surgery, pumped full of pain relief, I was encouraged to get out of bed and go to the bathroom under my own steam, and unless there is some driving factor that prevents this being done, so will you. To be honest, it is a really good confirmation bending your knee is ok and nothing is going to fall apart. After that, for the first week, the team doesn't want you to be moving around too much. But if you want to be able to sleep easily at night and get your prescribed exercise done each day, it is important you take what pain relief is recommended for you.

By reducing the pain you are experiencing, you allow your body the opportunity to start recovering instead of fighting your pain levels. We want your internal systems working the problem you want fixed most. Your new knee.

COMPLICATIONS

It should be a no-brainer—if any of the following occur, call your surgeon; if your surgeon is not available, get to your nearest GP or after-hours surgery:

- Body temperature exceeds 38.5 C / 101 F
- Shaking chills
- Severe pain or tenderness during activity and at rest
- Heavy bleeding from surgery incisions
- Pus or other liquids oozing from the incisions
- Bad smells from the wound when changing dressings
- Redness around the incision that is spreading
- Ongoing nausea or vomiting
- Decreasing ability to bend your leg
- A fall that results in reduced mobility
- Any concerns you may have

IF SOMETHING DOESN'T FEEL RIGHT—REACH OUT!

BLOOD THINNERS + ANTIBIOTICS

Because you won't be moving around very much for a couple of weeks, your surgeon may have prescribed a course of blood thinners, also known as anti-coagulants, as a clotting preventative. These are normally injected just under the skin in the stomach area.

I am not a fan of injecting myself, but I can do it when I have to, and initially, I would resort to numbing the area with a piece of ice first. When you have a cold therapy device in constant use—ice is always handy. But if you are not confident or squeamish and don't have someone to help you with this, your local chemist or visiting care person is generally happy to help out. My best friend is a nurse, and she loves the opportunity to jab me with a needle.

Remember, when you have finished the course of injectables, you can get rid of any spares and the needle bin at your local chemist. Don't just throw them in the bin.

If the hospital sent you home with antibiotics as well, then please take them until they are finished to ensure you don't get an infection post-surgery.

You don't get to leave the hospital without passing a multi-point physical.

As I have already mentioned, you have to have had a bowel movement before you leave, and if you have a board at the end of your bed with an empty checkbox for VOB—that stands for "voiding of the bowel"—it needs to be ticked before you leave. You don't have to show the nurse you "pooped," just make sure you tell them. Be prepared for questions on consistency and pain levels during the activity.

The exercises you have been given in the hospital will have to be completed to your physical therapist's satisfaction before your team will even consider sending you home.

For the last two days you are in the hospital, you will be on oral pain relief. Your team will be working with you to find the best combination of timings and medications that will reduce the pain sufficiently for you to complete your exercises properly.

Make a note of what timing works best for you so you can plan around this when you are back home.

MEDICATION TIMING AND IMPACT

BEDROOM ANTICS

Getting in and out of bed. You would think that is an easy thing to do. Well, it is, but not until you get shown the best way to do this activity with the least amount of pain.

Your nurse or physio will show you how to support your new knee with the foot on your OTHER leg to get in and out of bed. I didn't get shown this little trick until late into day two, and it was hard to get myself motivated enough to get out of bed to go to the bathroom each time until then as I knew it would hurt. But I still had to go. No bedpan for me.

Bedside cabinets hold all sorts of interesting stuff. Whilst you are recovering from your surgery, make room for your pain killers, lots of drinking water, your mobile phone, and charger. I have three mobile phone chargers setup around home: one each in my bedroom, office, and lounge. It isn't that I am lazy, but it isn't convenient to leave my phone on charge in my bedroom when I am working at the other end of the house in the office or my knee is too sore to get up off the couch.

What side of the bed do you sleep on? I used to be closest to the door, but I changed to the other side of the bed so that I was next to the wall. I found having a wall to support myself against while I tried to balance on my crutches when I got out of bed very handy. The blue glow from my phone charger light also provided just enough light to help me find my crutches in the middle of the night.

Turning over in bed is a challenge for the first couple of months. I literally had to wake up each time I wanted to roll over. A pillow between your legs might help, but your body will be keen to not hurt you, so you may end up with a bit of a sore back from sleeping in the same position all night.

You will be able to do some basic back stretching exercises once you are home, and a massage from a caring partner is always appropriate.

As to the other bedroom antics—that level of intimacy is totally between you and your partner. Whatever you can manage based on your pain levels and comfort. You may want to leave the Kama Sutra in the bottom drawer for a while longer.

THE WAY YOU WALK

There is a good chance the way you walk will be different after your surgery and when you finally ditch the crutches.

I have a lovely, crooked scar as my right leg was bowed prior to surgery due to the amount of cartilage removed over my various surgeries. Thank you, Sam, for making me less lopsided.

Once I was off crutches, my body had to adjust, and that meant a few visits to my chiropractor. Most health professionals have a bed that can take you from standing to lying down so you don't have to try to lift your knee up onto the adjustment table.

The surgery, your change of pace, your use of walking aids, and the changes to your knee will all impact your skeletal alignment. You should try to get in to see your preferred health practitioner for regular maintenance as soon as you can get to their clinic.

COLD THERAPY DEVICE—BEST THING SINCE SLICED BREAD

Sam, my surgeon, has a great setup where he includes the provision of a rental cold therapy unit as part of his service. This is an awesome recovery tool as it can reduce inflammation, swelling and nerve activity and will reduce your pain levels.

The cold therapy device was available to me as soon as I was out of surgery and awake enough to use it. I took full advantage of it being available. The nurses at my hospital were awesome; they would top up the ice for my machine day or night, just push the buzzer.

From an availability point of view, the hospital had a very large ice machine, so much like a pub, ice was always available. Your fridge might have an ice dispenser or you might have your own ice machine at home. I did buy a small ice maker; I found it on one of those "special of the day" internet sites, and it was in use constantly as it only put out three cups of ice at a time. We also have a chest freezer (bulk dog food) so my husband kept our freezer full so I could have ice any time I wanted. You can rent or buy a machine or just buy pre-bagged ice from somewhere locally as you need it.

If your surgeon doesn't offer a cold therapy unit as part of their service, you should be able to rent one through a local physiotherapist or purchase one of your own. I bought the Donjoy® Iceman with the universal pad (not included with the base unit), and at the time, the cost was approximately $250 AUD. If sports are a big part of your family life, purchasing your own cold therapy unit is not a bad idea and could save you money on future physiotherapy visits.

In the hospital you will be given exercises to complete daily over the next two weeks in the lead up to your wound review (performance review #1).

The physiotherapist will have specified the exact exercise, how many times to repeat the exercise (reps), and how many times a day (sessions) you should complete these.

Your day can very quickly get complicated when you combine these activities with taking your pain medications, antibiotics, blood thinners, icing your knee, and planning your day.

PLAN YOUR RECOVERY

Following the system I used, I have put together a daily plan and progress section so you can get yourself organised. Set a time each day to review your daily plan and track your own progress. It's hard to remember how you felt on a particular day, and if you wait too long to record it, you may forget bits. Your notes and planning info will be easy to find and can be reviewed by your surgeon and their team when you go back for your first review.

Some points on what you might want to track to make sure you are timing everything correctly:

- How do I feel overall?
- Am I tracking better this week than last?
- Pain level 1 hr before doing your exercises
- What medication and dosage did you take?
- At the time of completing your exercises:
    - Pain levels before exercise
    - How many reps and sessions did you do?
    - Pain levels after exercise
- Did you ice your knee after exercise?
- Did you achieve any of your goals today?
- Do you need to review your goals?

STAPLE HERE

- HOME EXERCISES GIVEN TO YOU AT THE HOSPITAL
- SHORT TERM MEDICATIONS LISTING

TIME	PLAN	ACTUAL
6:00 A.M.	TAKE MEDICATIONS	DONE
7:00 A.M.		
	BREATHE!	
8:00 A.M.	EXTENSIONS / BEND KNEE	ONLY DID 8 REPS ☹
	FOOT RAISE	10 DONE / ICED KNEE 1HR
9:00 A.M.	PAIN LEVELS?	6/10 ☹
10:00 A.M.	TAKE MEDICATIONS	DONE—PAIN 7/10 BEFORE ☹
11:00 A.M.	EXTENSIONS / BEND KNEE	DONE!
	FOOT RAISE	DONE! THEN ICED KNEE
12:00 P.M.		
	BREATHE	
1:00 P.M.	LUNCH	WASN'T HUNGRY
2:00 P.M.	TAKE MEDICATIONS	DONE—PAIN IS 8/10 ATM
3:00 P.M.	EXTENSIONS / BEND KNEE	MISSED—TOO SORE ☹
	FOOT RAISE	✓
4:00 P.M.	BREATHE	
5:00 P.M.		
	BREATHE	
6:00 P.M.	TAKE MEDICATIONS	DONE
7:00 P.M.	EXTENSIONS / BEND KNEE	10 DONE ☺
	FOOT RAISE	✓ ICED KNEE 1 HR
8:00 P.M.		
9:00 P.M.	BED	WENT @ 8:30—TIRED + SORE
10:00 P.M.		

DAY 1—REVIEW—EXAMPLE

ACTIVITY & SESSIONS/REPS	
EXTENSIONS	EXTEND LEG AND TRY TO STRAIGHTEN 10 REPS / 4X DAY
FOOT RAISE	PUSH KNEE DOWN AND TRY TO RAISE FOOT 10 REPS / 4X DAY
BREATHE!	10 BIG BREATHS
BEND KNEE	BEND KNEE—SEE NOTES 4 X DAY—WORK WITHIN PAIN LIMITS

NOTES / TO-DO LIST

How did you do today?

☑ BOOK CHIRO FOR SATURDAY

☑ ORDER NEXT WEEK'S MEALS

☐

☐

☐

☐

NOTES ABOUT TODAY

PAIN LEVELS WERE HORRIBLE TODAY—ONLY FIRST DAY AFTER SURGERY, SO I SLEPT A LOT AND DIDN'T EAT MUCH.

TIME	PLAN	ACTUAL
6:00 A.M.		
7:00 A.M.		
8:00 A.M.		
9:00 A.M.		
10:00 A.M.		
11:00 A.M.		
12:00 P.M.		
1:00 P.M.		
2:00 P.M.		
3:00 P.M.		
4:00 P.M.		
5:00 P.M.		
6:00 P.M.		
7:00 P.M.		
8:00 P.M.		
9:00 P.M.		
10:00 P.M.		

DAY 1—REVIEW

ACTIVITY & SESSIONS/REPS	

NOTES / TO-DO LIST

How did you do today?

☐

☐

☐

☐

☐

☐

☐

NOTES ABOUT TODAY

TIME	PLAN	ACTUAL
6:00 A.M.		
7:00 A.M.		
8:00 A.M.		
9:00 A.M.		
10:00 A.M.		
11:00 A.M.		
12:00 P.M.		
1:00 P.M.		
2:00 P.M.		
3:00 P.M.		
4:00 P.M.		
5:00 P.M.		
6:00 P.M.		
7:00 P.M.		
8:00 P.M.		
9:00 P.M.		
10:00 P.M.		

ACTIVITY & SESSIONS/REPS	

NOTES / TO-DO LIST

How did you do today?

- ☐
- ☐
- ☐
- ☐
- ☐
- ☐
- ☐

NOTES ABOUT TODAY

TIME	PLAN	ACTUAL
6:00 A.M.		
7:00 A.M.		
8:00 A.M.		
9:00 A.M.		
10:00 A.M.		
11:00 A.M.		
12:00 P.M.		
1:00 P.M.		
2:00 P.M.		
3:00 P.M.		
4:00 P.M.		
5:00 P.M.		
6:00 P.M.		
7:00 P.M.		
8:00 P.M.		
9:00 P.M.		
10:00 P.M.		

ACTIVITY & SESSIONS/REPS	

NOTES / TO-DO LIST

How did you do today?

☐

☐

☐

☐

☐

☐

☐

NOTES ABOUT TODAY

TIME	PLAN	ACTUAL
6:00 A.M.		
7:00 A.M.		
8:00 A.M.		
9:00 A.M.		
10:00 A.M.		
11:00 A.M.		
12:00 P.M.		
1:00 P.M.		
2:00 P.M.		
3:00 P.M.		
4:00 P.M.		
5:00 P.M.		
6:00 P.M.		
7:00 P.M.		
8:00 P.M.		
9:00 P.M.		
10:00 P.M.		

ACTIVITY & SESSIONS/REPS	

NOTES / TO-DO LIST

How did you do today?

- ☐
- ☐
- ☐
- ☐
- ☐
- ☐
- ☐

NOTES ABOUT TODAY

TIME	PLAN	ACTUAL
6:00 A.M.		
7:00 A.M.		
8:00 A.M.		
9:00 A.M.		
10:00 A.M.		
11:00 A.M.		
12:00 P.M.		
1:00 P.M.		
2:00 P.M.		
3:00 P.M.		
4:00 P.M.		
5:00 P.M.		
6:00 P.M.		
7:00 P.M.		
8:00 P.M.		
9:00 P.M.		
10:00 P.M.		

ACTIVITY & SESSIONS/REPS	

NOTES / TO-DO LIST

How did you do today?

☐

☐

☐

☐

☐

☐

☐

NOTES ABOUT TODAY

TIME	PLAN	ACTUAL
6:00 A.M.		
7:00 A.M.		
8:00 A.M.		
9:00 A.M.		
10:00 A.M.		
11:00 A.M.		
12:00 P.M.		
1:00 P.M.		
2:00 P.M.		
3:00 P.M.		
4:00 P.M.		
5:00 P.M.		
6:00 P.M.		
7:00 P.M.		
8:00 P.M.		
9:00 P.M.		
10:00 P.M.		

DAY 6—REVIEW

How did you do today?

☐

☐

☐

☐

☐

☐

☐

NOTES ABOUT TODAY

TIME	PLAN	ACTUAL
6:00 A.M.		
7:00 A.M.		
8:00 A.M.		
9:00 A.M.		
10:00 A.M.		
11:00 A.M.		
12:00 P.M.		
1:00 P.M.		
2:00 P.M.		
3:00 P.M.		
4:00 P.M.		
5:00 P.M.		
6:00 P.M.		
7:00 P.M.		
8:00 P.M.		
9:00 P.M.		
10:00 P.M.		

ACTIVITY & SESSIONS/REPS	

NOTES / TO-DO LIST

How did you do today?

☐

☐

☐

☐

☐

☐

☐

NOTES ABOUT TODAY

TIME	PLAN	ACTUAL
6:00 A.M.		
7:00 A.M.		
8:00 A.M.		
9:00 A.M.		
10:00 A.M.		
11:00 A.M.		
12:00 P.M.		
1:00 P.M.		
2:00 P.M.		
3:00 P.M.		
4:00 P.M.		
5:00 P.M.		
6:00 P.M.		
7:00 P.M.		
8:00 P.M.		
9:00 P.M.		
10:00 P.M.		

ACTIVITY & SESSIONS/REPS

NOTES ABOUT TODAY

NOTES / TO-DO LIST

How did you do today?

☐

☐

☐

☐

☐

☐

TIME	PLAN	ACTUAL
6:00 A.M.		
7:00 A.M.		
8:00 A.M.		
9:00 A.M.		
10:00 A.M.		
11:00 A.M.		
12:00 P.M.		
1:00 P.M.		
2:00 P.M.		
3:00 P.M.		
4:00 P.M.		
5:00 P.M.		
6:00 P.M.		
7:00 P.M.		
8:00 P.M.		
9:00 P.M.		
10:00 P.M.		

ACTIVITY & SESSIONS/REPS	

NOTES / TO-DO LIST

How did you do today?

☐

☐

☐

☐

☐

☐

☐

NOTES ABOUT TODAY

TIME	PLAN	ACTUAL
6:00 A.M.		
7:00 A.M.		
8:00 A.M.		
9:00 A.M.		
10:00 A.M.		
11:00 A.M.		
12:00 P.M.		
1:00 P.M.		
2:00 P.M.		
3:00 P.M.		
4:00 P.M.		
5:00 P.M.		
6:00 P.M.		
7:00 P.M.		
8:00 P.M.		
9:00 P.M.		
10:00 P.M.		

ACTIVITY & SESSIONS/REPS	

NOTES / TO-DO LIST

How did you do today?

- [ ]
- [ ]
- [ ]
- [ ]
- [ ]
- [ ]
- [ ]

NOTES ABOUT TODAY

TIME	PLAN	ACTUAL
6:00 A.M.		
7:00 A.M.		
8:00 A.M.		
9:00 A.M.		
10:00 A.M.		
11:00 A.M.		
12:00 P.M.		
1:00 P.M.		
2:00 P.M.		
3:00 P.M.		
4:00 P.M.		
5:00 P.M.		
6:00 P.M.		
7:00 P.M.		
8:00 P.M.		
9:00 P.M.		
10:00 P.M.		

ACTIVITY & SESSIONS/REPS	

NOTES / TO-DO LIST

How did you do today?

☐

☐

☐

☐

☐

☐

☐

NOTES ABOUT TODAY

TIME	PLAN	ACTUAL
6:00 A.M.		
7:00 A.M.		
8:00 A.M.		
9:00 A.M.		
10:00 A.M.		
11:00 A.M.		
12:00 P.M.		
1:00 P.M.		
2:00 P.M.		
3:00 P.M.		
4:00 P.M.		
5:00 P.M.		
6:00 P.M.		
7:00 P.M.		
8:00 P.M.		
9:00 P.M.		
10:00 P.M.		

ACTIVITY & SESSIONS/REPS	

NOTES / TO-DO LIST

How did you do today?

☐

☐

☐

☐

☐

☐

☐

NOTES ABOUT TODAY

TIME	PLAN	ACTUAL
6:00 A.M.		
7:00 A.M.		
8:00 A.M.		
9:00 A.M.		
10:00 A.M.		
11:00 A.M.		
12:00 P.M.		
1:00 P.M.		
2:00 P.M.		
3:00 P.M.		
4:00 P.M.		
5:00 P.M.		
6:00 P.M.		
7:00 P.M.		
8:00 P.M.		
9:00 P.M.		
10:00 P.M.		

ACTIVITY & SESSIONS/REPS	

NOTES / TO-DO LIST

How did you do today?

☐

☐

☐

☐

☐

☐

☐

NOTES ABOUT TODAY

TIME	PLAN	ACTUAL
6:00 A.M.		
7:00 A.M.		
8:00 A.M.		
9:00 A.M.		
10:00 A.M.		
11:00 A.M.		
12:00 P.M.		
1:00 P.M.		
2:00 P.M.		
3:00 P.M.		
4:00 P.M.		
5:00 P.M.		
6:00 P.M.		
7:00 P.M.		
8:00 P.M.		
9:00 P.M.		
10:00 P.M.		

DAY 14—REVIEW

ACTIVITY & SESSIONS/REPS	

NOTES / TO-DO LIST

How did you do today?

☐

☐

☐

☐

☐

☐

☐

NOTES ABOUT TODAY

DAY SPARE—PLAN

TIME	PLAN	ACTUAL
6:00 A.M.		
7:00 A.M.		
8:00 A.M.		
9:00 A.M.		
10:00 A.M.		
11:00 A.M.		
12:00 P.M.		
1:00 P.M.		
2:00 P.M.		
3:00 P.M.		
4:00 P.M.		
5:00 P.M.		
6:00 P.M.		
7:00 P.M.		
8:00 P.M.		
9:00 P.M.		
10:00 P.M.		

DAY SPARE—REVIEW

<table>
<tr><td>ACTIVITY & SESSIONS/REPS</td><td>NOTES / TO-DO LIST</td></tr>
</table>

How did you do today?

☐

☐

☐

☐

☐

☐

☐

NOTES ABOUT TODAY

DAY SPARE—PLAN

TIME	PLAN	ACTUAL
6:00 A.M.		
7:00 A.M.		
8:00 A.M.		
9:00 A.M.		
10:00 A.M.		
11:00 A.M.		
12:00 P.M.		
1:00 P.M.		
2:00 P.M.		
3:00 P.M.		
4:00 P.M.		
5:00 P.M.		
6:00 P.M.		
7:00 P.M.		
8:00 P.M.		
9:00 P.M.		
10:00 P.M.		

ACTIVITY & SESSIONS/REPS	

NOTES / TO-DO LIST

How did you do today?

☐

☐

☐

☐

☐

☐

☐

NOTES ABOUT TODAY

DAY SPARE—PLAN

TIME	PLAN	ACTUAL
6:00 A.M.		
7:00 A.M.		
8:00 A.M.		
9:00 A.M.		
10:00 A.M.		
11:00 A.M.		
12:00 P.M.		
1:00 P.M.		
2:00 P.M.		
3:00 P.M.		
4:00 P.M.		
5:00 P.M.		
6:00 P.M.		
7:00 P.M.		
8:00 P.M.		
9:00 P.M.		
10:00 P.M.		

ACTIVITY & SESSIONS/REPS	

NOTES / TO-DO LIST

How did you do today?

- ☐
- ☐
- ☐
- ☐
- ☐
- ☐
- ☐

NOTES ABOUT TODAY

2 WEEKS POST SURGERY

Approximately two weeks after surgery, you will be heading back to the surgeon's offices to have your wound reviewed and a progress check on how you are going with your rehabilitation exercises—Performance Review #1.

So long as you have been following your plan and doing your exercises with the correct level of pain relief, this visit shouldn't result in any surprises.

Your surgeon or the nurse will remove any stitches or staples (if you had any), review your ability to bend and straighten your knee, ability to complete exercises, and review your pain management requirements.

If you are on track, you will be booked in for another performance review in six weeks. Well done, you!

At this point in your recovery, your surgeon will encourage you to find a local physiotherapist, physical therapist, or carer service who will work with you on additional exercises. These will replace or expand your current exercise program and are designed to improve your strength, stability, and range of motion. If you have had some challenges with the exercises given to you at the hospital, you may have to continue with your current exercise regime and will be booked in for an additional review in a couple of weeks.

If you have done exceptionally well you can ask, but it is unlikely you will get a yes just yet, to driving. Your surgeon will advise what they want to see from you before you are cleared to drive again.

Usually, the caveat is you must be off the serious pain relief and able to get around without your crutches.

A gentle reminder your motor vehicle insurance company may not cover you if you drive before being cleared and have an accident.

For the next four weeks, your goal is to ditch the crutches and reduce your pain medication to just paracetamol when doing your exercises.

SCAR MANAGEMENT—ASK AN EXPERT

It's not that cool to have a massive scar that looks like someone went at your leg with a hack saw and you got sewn back together by the vet.

With a little care, you can make sure your scar is nearly invisible. Take the time to research scar treatments available as there are new solutions coming onto the market every year. I find the best advice is usually from a company that deals with scars all the time. For me it was my local skin cancer clinic, but plastic surgeons have great resources too, as they deal with scars on a daily basis. Either will know what they are talking about and give you good advice.

PHYSICAL THERAPIST—AKA PERSONAL TORTURER

Over the next four to six weeks, you will be working with your chosen physical therapist to increase the range of movement you already have and increase your confidence getting around the house without your crutches.

This is the hard part of the process as your knee will NOT feel stable, and going out in public can be very daunting and extremely tiring. If you have graduated from crutches at home, but still a bit wobbly, take just one with you when you go out. Once I got off crutches altogether, I would find a shopping trolley as soon as I got out of my car and use it as support from the car park into the shopping centre and back again—perfect to support you and make sure people don't knock you around.

Be prepared to sit down and take a break mid-shopping, and mostly, be patient with yourself, continue to ice your knee, and do the exercises as advised by your physical therapist.

Document daily how you are going with your pain levels, when your appointments are booked with your health professionals, and how you are tracking with completing your exercises with the pain medications you ARE taking.

KEY PERFORMANCE INDICATORS

Now is the time to get creative but still remain realistic about what goals you need to achieve in the next six weeks that will let you ditch the crutches and get on with your life!

WEEK 1

WEEK 2

WEEK 3

WEEK 4

WEEK 5

WEEK 6

Staple any handouts and notes you get from your personal torture therapist here.

	6 A.M.	8 A.M.	10 A.M.	NOON	2 P.M.	4 P.M.	6 P.M.	8 P.M.	10 P.M.
MONDAY NOTES:									
PLAN									
ACTUAL									
REVIEW									
TUESDAY NOTES:									
PLAN									
ACTUAL									
REVIEW									
WEDNESDAY NOTES:									
PLAN									
ACTUAL									
REVIEW									
THURSDAY NOTES:									
PLAN									
ACTUAL									
REVIEW									
FRIDAY NOTES:									
PLAN									
ACTUAL									
REVIEW									
SATURDAY NOTES:									
PLAN									
ACTUAL									
REVIEW									
SUNDAY NOTES:									
PLAN									
ACTUAL									
REVIEW									

WEEK 1—REVIEW IT

<table>
<tr><td colspan="2">ACTIVITY & SESSIONS/REPS</td><td>NOTES / TO-DO LIST</td></tr>
<tr><td></td><td></td><td>Fail to Plan, Plan to Fail!</td></tr>
<tr><td></td><td></td><td>☐</td></tr>
<tr><td></td><td></td><td>☐</td></tr>
<tr><td></td><td></td><td>☐</td></tr>
<tr><td></td><td></td><td>☐</td></tr>
<tr><td></td><td></td><td>☐</td></tr>
<tr><td></td><td></td><td>☐</td></tr>
<tr><td></td><td></td><td>☐</td></tr>
</table>

WEEK 1 IN REVIEW:

	6 A.M.	8 A.M.	10 A.M.	NOON	2 P.M.	4 P.M.	6 P.M.	8 P.M.	10 P.M.
MONDAY NOTES:									
PLAN									
ACTUAL									
REVIEW									
TUESDAY NOTES:									
PLAN									
ACTUAL									
REVIEW									
WEDNESDAY NOTES:									
PLAN									
ACTUAL									
REVIEW									
THURSDAY NOTES:									
PLAN									
ACTUAL									
REVIEW									
FRIDAY NOTES:									
PLAN									
ACTUAL									
REVIEW									
SATURDAY NOTES:									
PLAN									
ACTUAL									
REVIEW									
SUNDAY NOTES:									
PLAN									
ACTUAL									
REVIEW									

WEEK 2—REVIEW IT

ACTIVITY & SESSIONS/REPS	

NOTES / TO-DO LIST
Fail to Plan, Plan to Fail!
☐
☐
☐
☐
☐
☐
☐

WEEK 2 IN REVIEW:

I hope you got a gold star from your personal torture therapist this week. ☺

Did they issue more exercises for you to do?

Staple any handouts and notes you get from your personal torture therapist here.

	6 A.M.	8 A.M.	10 A.M.	NOON	2 P.M.	4 P.M.	6 P.M.	8 P.M.	10 P.M.
MONDAY NOTES:									
PLAN									
ACTUAL									
REVIEW									
TUESDAY NOTES:									
PLAN									
ACTUAL									
REVIEW									
WEDNESDAY NOTES:									
PLAN									
ACTUAL									
REVIEW									
THURSDAY NOTES:									
PLAN									
ACTUAL									
REVIEW									
FRIDAY NOTES:									
PLAN									
ACTUAL									
REVIEW									
SATURDAY NOTES:									
PLAN									
ACTUAL									
REVIEW									
SUNDAY NOTES:									
PLAN									
ACTUAL									
REVIEW									

ACTIVITY & SESSIONS/REPS	

NOTES / TO-DO LIST

Fail to Plan, Plan to Fail!

- [ ]
- [ ]
- [ ]
- [ ]
- [ ]
- [ ]
- [ ]

WEEK 3 IN REVIEW:

	6 A.M.	8 A.M.	10 A.M.	NOON	2 P.M.	4 P.M.	6 P.M.	8 P.M.	10 P.M.
MONDAY NOTES:									
PLAN									
ACTUAL									
REVIEW									
TUESDAY NOTES:									
PLAN									
ACTUAL									
REVIEW									
WEDNESDAY NOTES:									
PLAN									
ACTUAL									
REVIEW									
THURSDAY NOTES:									
PLAN									
ACTUAL									
REVIEW									
FRIDAY NOTES:									
PLAN									
ACTUAL									
REVIEW									
SATURDAY NOTES:									
PLAN									
ACTUAL									
REVIEW									
SUNDAY NOTES:									
PLAN									
ACTUAL									
REVIEW									

WEEK 4—REVIEW IT

ACTIVITY & SESSIONS/REPS	

NOTES / TO-DO LIST

Fail to Plan, Plan to Fail!

- ☐
- ☐
- ☐
- ☐
- ☐
- ☐
- ☐

WEEK 4 IN REVIEW:

You should be well on your way to getting rid of your crutches!

Your physical therapy should be showing results. Remember how little you could do when you first got out of surgery—be happy with your results; you are being awesome and taking control of your results.

Any new information or exercises from your physical therapist?

Staple them here so you can find them when you need them.

	6 A.M.	8 A.M.	10 A.M.	NOON	2 P.M.	4 P.M.	6 P.M.	8 P.M.	10 P.M.
MONDAY NOTES:									
PLAN									
ACTUAL									
REVIEW									
TUESDAY NOTES:									
PLAN									
ACTUAL									
REVIEW									
WEDNESDAY NOTES:									
PLAN									
ACTUAL									
REVIEW									
THURSDAY NOTES:									
PLAN									
ACTUAL									
REVIEW									
FRIDAY NOTES:									
PLAN									
ACTUAL									
REVIEW									
SATURDAY NOTES:									
PLAN									
ACTUAL									
REVIEW									
SUNDAY NOTES:									
PLAN									
ACTUAL									
REVIEW									

WEEK 5—REVIEW IT

ACTIVITY & SESSIONS/REPS	

NOTES / TO-DO LIST

☐

☐

☐

☐

☐

☐

☐

WEEK 5 IN REVIEW:

	6 A.M.	8 A.M.	10 A.M.	NOON	2 P.M.	4 P.M.	6 P.M.	8 P.M.	10 P.M.
MONDAY NOTES:									
PLAN									
ACTUAL									
REVIEW									
TUESDAY NOTES:									
PLAN									
ACTUAL									
REVIEW									
WEDNESDAY NOTES:									
PLAN									
ACTUAL									
REVIEW									
THURSDAY NOTES:									
PLAN									
ACTUAL									
REVIEW									
FRIDAY NOTES:									
PLAN									
ACTUAL									
REVIEW									
SATURDAY NOTES:									
PLAN									
ACTUAL									
REVIEW									
SUNDAY NOTES:									
PLAN									
ACTUAL									
REVIEW									

WEEK 6—REVIEW IT

ACTIVITY & SESSIONS/REPS	

NOTES / TO-DO LIST
Fail to Plan, Plan to Fail!
☐
☐
☐
☐
☐
☐
☐

WEEK 6 IN REVIEW:

Your physical therapist may be around for a while still, so even though you may be cleared to drive and your surgeon doesn't want to see you for another six months, you might still have more work to do.

Staple your handouts here and refer back to them as you need.

UNHIRE EQUIPMENT

Time to return some of your medical aids if you are not using them anymore.

Don't forget to lodge a claim with your private health for the cost of your post-surgery medical aids, if you are covered.

	6 A.M.	8 A.M.	10 A.M.	NOON	2 P.M.	4 P.M.	6 P.M.	8 P.M.	10 P.M.
MONDAY NOTES:									
PLAN									
ACTUAL									
REVIEW									
TUESDAY NOTES:									
PLAN									
ACTUAL									
REVIEW									
WEDNESDAY NOTES:									
PLAN									
ACTUAL									
REVIEW									
THURSDAY NOTES:									
PLAN									
ACTUAL									
REVIEW									
FRIDAY NOTES:									
PLAN									
ACTUAL									
REVIEW									
SATURDAY NOTES:									
PLAN									
ACTUAL									
REVIEW									
SUNDAY NOTES:									
PLAN									
ACTUAL									
REVIEW									

WEEK 7—REVIEW IT

ACTIVITY & SESSIONS/REPS	

Fail to Plan, Plan to Fail!

☐

☐

☐

☐

☐

☐

☐

WEEK 7 IN REVIEW:

	6 A.M.	8 A.M.	10 A.M.	NOON	2 P.M.	4 P.M.	6 P.M.	8 P.M.	10 P.M.
MONDAY NOTES:									
PLAN									
ACTUAL									
REVIEW									
TUESDAY NOTES:									
PLAN									
ACTUAL									
REVIEW									
WEDNESDAY NOTES:									
PLAN									
ACTUAL									
REVIEW									
THURSDAY NOTES:									
PLAN									
ACTUAL									
REVIEW									
FRIDAY NOTES:									
PLAN									
ACTUAL									
REVIEW									
SATURDAY NOTES:									
PLAN									
ACTUAL									
REVIEW									
SUNDAY NOTES:									
PLAN									
ACTUAL									
REVIEW									

ACTIVITY & SESSIONS/REPS	

NOTES / TO-DO LIST

Fail to Plan, Plan to Fail!

☐

☐

☐

☐

☐

☐

☐

WEEK 8 IN REVIEW:

DITCH THE CRUTCHES

By now you should be comfortable enough to be using maybe just a single crutch when going outside and should be able get around slowly by yourself around the house without crutches at all.

Don't be too hard on yourself; be patient with your recovery. You may not be as mobile as you might like, but your knee is probably still swollen and you are going to continue to ice it for the next few weeks to support the healing process. Thank goodness for the cold therapy device!

It's going to take some time for your body to adjust to your new knee (my new knee is still much hotter to touch than the other, and I am more than three months post-surgery).

CLEARED TO DRIVE

If you have done the work, your surgeon should be giving you the all clear to get back behind the wheel and back to menacing the other drivers on the road.

When parking, make sure you give yourself enough room to get yourself in and out of the car without bending your knee too much, if you are eligible for a parking permit that gives you access to better and wider parking spots—use it!

6 WEEK GOAL REVIEW	ACHIEVED?

THE NEXT 6 MONTHS

You planned and worked your first six weeks of recovery.

This is the hardest part of your recovery done and dusted.

However, for the next six months, you still have work to do to get your knee to where you can do all of the things you want to get back to.

Most likely you will still be visiting your physical therapist for a few more months.

You will still need some help around the house and gardens. It was a minimum of three months before I could do any gardening, and I needed to sit on a small stool when doing weeding and planting out my garlic for the season.

So don't tell the lawn mowing man to stop coming around just yet. Do start planning what you want to achieve in the next six months.

Will you do the work to achieve your goals?

MONTH 1—I CAN DRIVE AGAIN (IF I WANT TO)!

ACTIVITY & SESSIONS/REPS	

NOTES / TO-DO LIST

Where to put my crutches in the car?

☐

☐

☐

☐

☐

☐

☐

MONTH 1 IN REVIEW:

MONTH 2—GO SHOPPING BY YOURSELF!

ACTIVITY & SESSIONS/REPS	

NOTES / TO-DO LIST

I can go to the shops!

☐

☐

☐

☐

☐

☐

☐

MONTH 2 IN REVIEW:

ACTIVITY & SESSIONS/REPS		NOTES / TO-DO LIST
		Look, Mum—no hands!
		☐
		☐
		☐
		☐
		☐
		☐
		☐

MONTH 3 IN REVIEW:

MONTH 4—DOG WALKING IS BACK ON!

ACTIVITY & SESSIONS/REPS	

NOTES / TO-DO LIST

Walking the dogs!

☐

☐

☐

☐

☐

☐

☐

MONTH 4 IN REVIEW:

MONTH 5—KNEE NO LONGER FEELS WOBBLY!

ACTIVITY & SESSIONS/REPS	

NOTES / TO-DO LIST

☐

☐

☐

☐

☐

☐

☐

MONTH 5 IN REVIEW:

MONTH 6—NEARLY BACK TO NORMAL!

ACTIVITY & SESSIONS/REPS	

NOTES / TO-DO LIST

Get ready for clearance to live!

☐ CONFIRM SURGEON APPOINTMENT FOR PERFORMANCE REVIEW #3!

☐

☐

☐

☐

☐

☐

MONTH 6 IN REVIEW:

6 MONTHS POST-SURGERY

So I am really hoping you passed your third performance review with flying colours like I did.

This last consult with your surgeon should have been a review on what went well for you and what you can expect now you are cleared to get on with the rest of your life. Yah, for you!

Remember how back on one of the early pages of this book you wrote down your pain points? I asked you to document all the things you couldn't do before your knee surgery and because of the osteoarthritic damage to your knee.

Maybe you wrote them down; maybe you didn't.

Your replacement knee may not be completely the same as the one you had twenty years ago, but it will be close enough to give you back some quality of life. If you go back now and look at the daily activities you couldn't do because of the pain you were in I hope you are back on track and looking to take those activities up again, if you haven't already.

I sincerely hope this book has provided you with some useful tips and tricks you have been able to use to get you through your own journey.

Since this book was first envisioned, I have had a lumbar fusion of the spine—also another common osteoarthritic surgery—and my mum has had a hip replacement. These are just food for more books, so if you have either of these coming up, look me up for where you can grab another guide. Each surgery has different preparation and recovery plans.

I know I may have missed some things from this book that you may have experienced. If you think of anything that you feel could be added to a future version of ths book, then please write them down on the next page, and if you can scan or take a picture of your suggestions and email them to me, I would love to incorporate them into the next version.

I would love to hear of your success and how the book fitted your recovery.

You can go to my website to leave a review of the book or send me some feedback if you feel like typing it up.

Thank you and get back to fun with your new knee.

Katy

You can email me at tkr@katyvincent.com